Beginners Intuitive Eating Guide

The Anti-Diet Guide to Stop Chronic Dieting, Make Peace with Food, & Love Yourself.

Eiden Raven

circumstances is the author responsible for any losses, direct or indirect, that are incurred as a result of the use of the information contained within this document, including, but not limited to, errors, omissions, or inaccuracies.

Table of Contents

Introduction

Trying to be healthy is becoming more and more confusing. We are bombarded with all types of diets, metabolic profiles that supposedly link with specific exercise regimes and how to ratio your macros, and social media accounts everywhere of girls and women who have tiny waists, huge muscular thighs, and who make everything they eat with protein powder. This just doesn't seem natural—from the way people look to the concoctions that they eat. How did society end up here? What happened to the days when you could just eat a cookie, forget about it, and get on with your day?

Being fit and healthy is extremely important, especially because most of us live a sedentary lifestyle; however, I think that there's a middle ground here. Following a specific eating pattern or diet is a form of restriction, and I sometimes wonder why people need these restrictive rules in their lives. What became of eating when you know your body needs it, and stopping when you know your body has had enough? Accordingly, if your body doesn't need food, you don't eat any. Isn't that what our ancestors used to do? Because eating and food have become such an integral part of our lives, practicing intuitive eating or developing an intuitive eating mentality is hard, we're not only pressured by friends and family to eat when they eat, we're also constantly surrounded by food, and food has become the center point of most social activities.

Intuitive eating is knowing when your body needs nourishment and living without restrictions. In this guide, we are going to look at mindful eating as well. Mindful eating is different from intuitive eating in some senses and similar in others. However, intuitive eating provides total freedom when it comes to food choices, but in some cases, when you are so far removed from your body's natural impulses and responses, using mindful eating to bring you back to that point where you are able to connect with your body's natural signals and impulses can be very useful.

In the end, you can expect numerous benefits from intuitive eating, and although the journey may be a challenging one because it requires a change in one's state of mind, the end result and health you experience after finally 'getting' your body, what it needs, and how much it needs are mind-blowing. Here are some of the research-based benefits you can get from adopting an intuitive eating lifestyle (apart from some real sanity):

- A higher level of satisfaction with life.
- A natural sense of wellbeing and optimism.
- Dramatically reduced cases of emotional eating.
- Virtually no chance of developing any form of disordered eating.
- A sense of proactivity in your approach to life and coping.
- Higher levels of 'good' cholesterol. Lowered levels of Triglyceride.
- A better relationship with your body and body image.
- High self-esteem.

These effects have been noted in over 100 studies conducted about intuitive eating. You develop these health benefits because you start experiencing a sense of freedom that you never thought could be coupled with health and a healthy body image (Rumsey, 2019).

Intuitive Eating has 10 important principles that will not only help you to understand the practice in itself, but will also serve as a guide to lead you to the point where you can practice intuitive eating without any concerns. These principles all emphasize the unconditional freedom one needs to experience and how this should be closely linked with your body's needs and not your emotional needs. In each chapter, we will discuss one principle and will explain each principle within the context of the chapter's subject to help us understand the big picture of intuitive eating, why it may take some time to truly release yourself from the shackles of diet culture, and what it may take to stand up for your own freedom, physically and mentally, in order to be the most fulfilled, healthiest, and happiest individual you can be.

This is your time. The time to get to know and understand your body is now. Embrace it and enjoy the journey.

Chapter 1: The Intuitive Eating Lowdown

One of the best ways to define intuitive eating is "the dynamic process-integrating attunement of mind, body, and food" (The Original Intuitive Eating Pros, 2021). This definition illustrates what separates intuitive eating from other 'diets' and eating patterns that claim to promote health and weight loss. Intuitive eating is quite literally the integration of the body, mind, and of food. In other words, the sole purpose of food is to keep the mind and the body healthy and happy, and one way of doing that is to take away eating restrictions and allow the body to tell the mind when you need to eat and when the body has had enough nourishment. To some, this may sound like an excuse to binge on your favorite foods all day; however, when you've reached the point where your mind is free from that obsession with food, the thought of constantly eating when your body does not need the nutrients will not make any sense to you. So, if you want to learn about intuitive eating, where should you start?

What Is Intuitive Eating?

Something that baffles people about intuitive eaters and the fact that they are usually healthy and in good shape is that intuitive eating is an anti-diet approach. To become an intuitive eater, you need to go on a journey to get to know your body and your mind, tune into what kind of nourishment your body needs, and understand signals like hunger, fullness, and satisfaction. Most importantly, intuitive eating means that you trust your body (and your mind) to be around food without having any rules about how to approach situations involving food. Instead of drooling, you are dismissively neutral. "Oh, *hors d'oeuvres* again? How quaint. Unfortunately, I'm not hungry right now." Alternatively, it could go down this way, "Oh, *hors d'oeuvres* again? I'm a bit peckish, let me have one." If you were to go into that room where all these lovely platters were floating around but you have pre-established rules and restrictions about food in your head, one of two things is likely to happen: you will either suffer the whole time because you know you are not allowed to touch any of the yummy snacks and will leave feeling frustrated and depraved, or you'll take a plate and pile it sky-high with *hors d'oeuvres,* consume them all, and feel terrible because your body didn't actually need any of that food.

Intuitive eating is a tool to help you to live your life unapologetically and to ditch the guilt surrounding food. Ironically, intuitive eating is a concept created by two dietitians named Elyse Resch and Evelyn Tribole in 1995. Their approach is to not focus on restrictions or rules when it comes to healthy eating, but rather, to focus on behavioral aspects. Their idea extends back to icons like Susie Orbach, who, in 1978, authored the book *Fat is a Feminist Idea.* Another advocate of this approach is Geneen Roth, a famous figure who has been writing about the concept of emotional eating since the early 1980s. Even before that, a weight management program loosely based on intuitive eating was founded by Thelma Wayler in 1972 called *Green Mountain at Fox Run,* which was based in Vermont. As you can see, the idea of this natural approach has existed for years alongside the development of diet culture; however, intuitive eating gained prominence contemporarily, especially due to the fact that diet culture has taken such an extremist and confusing direction (Jennings, 2019).

Aren't we all born with intuition about when we need to eat and when not? A baby will not feed on their mother or take a bite of food if they are not hungry. Somewhere, as we grew up, our relationship with food becomes distorted; intuitive eating aims to restore the natural relationship we have with food and free us from our restrictions.

Studies conducted on intuitive eaters have found that intuitive eating has positive nutritional benefits because intuitive eaters are not bound to any restrictive diets and, therefore, are more likely to consume a variety of foods that tick all the boxes of their nutritional profile. In other words, intuitive eaters are more likely to get balanced nutritional benefits from their way of eating (Dutta, 2019).

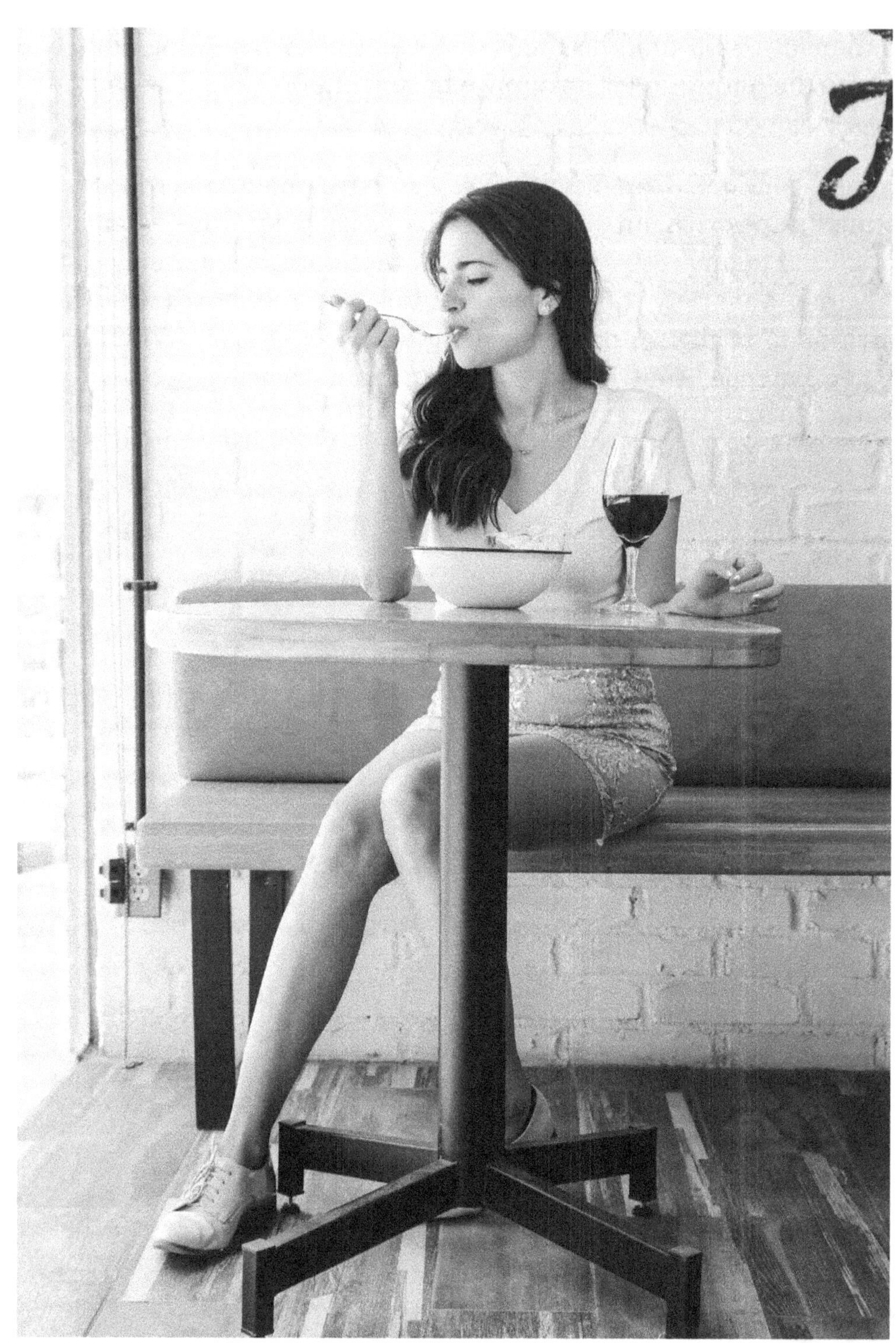

Research on intuitive eating is mostly conducted on women, possibly because women are more likely to be caught in the web of diet culture. Women are also more likely to develop misinformed eating habits, distorted body images, and end up restricting themselves which can have mental repercussions. It is not surprising that researchers have found one of the biggest benefits of intuitive eating to be better psychological health. I suspect that this benefit is related to the sense of freedom you feel when you develop a sense of intuitive eating.

Other fantastic benefits of this approach include a lower body mass index, or BMI, a positive outlook, and an increased ability to manage your weight. One study conducted in 2012 indicated that women who scored high on the intuitive eating scale also had significantly lower body mass index levels; this strongly suggests that if the only reason you tend to eat is in response to your body's hunger and satiety cues and not for any recreational, emotional, or social purposes - even though you have unconditional freedom to eat, you are unlikely to develop eating behaviors that will lead to weight gain (The Original Intuitive Eating Pros, 2021). Participants of another study about intuitive eating reported experiencing less anxiety and decreased levels of depression. One study, after observing women's eating behavior and eating patterns, reported that women who tend to eat intuitively are less likely to develop a disordered form of eating because disordered eating is based on restrictions and a sense of control (Jennings, 2019).

Intuitive Eating: The Principles

Most experts on intuitive eating will tell you that, to understand intuitive eating, you need to understand the 10 principles that support and define intuitive eating. In each chapter, we'll be touching on one of the principles. The first, very important principle of intuitive eating is to honor your health.

Principle 1: Honor Your Hunger

Eating, and deciding what and when to eat, has become a bizarre battle between body and mind. The mind, in most cases, has shut off signals coming from the body, which means that even though you think you are making the correct decisions about food, your body likely doesn't have a say in this. In an ideal world, health must come before physical appearance, but what makes our lives even more bizarre is how distorted "healthy" physical attributes have become. I've made the mistake of clicking on an Instagram profile of a health and fitness influencer and subsequently receiving countless emails that provide tidbits of fitness and nutritional advice in order to get me to purchase one of the influencer's programs. Is making donuts, pancakes, and muffins from Whey protein powder going to make me healthier? Also, is doing wild plyometric exercises using kettlebells going to help me become who I want to be? There are so many health and fitness influencers out there, but blindly following them is not the answer. To honor your health, you have to know what it means for your body to be healthy. You also need to connect your body and your mind so that you can take the piles of information that are hauled at you every day when you go onto social media, and must understand which of these 'hacks' will work for you and which of them won't.

Health is not an "all or nothing" idea, moderation is definitely most beneficial for the mind and body. In other words, being healthy doesn't mean you have to have the perfect eating habits all of the time—you just need your body to regulate them naturally and make suggestions that will end up being most beneficial for your health. Embrace the idea of gentle nutrition, where food is not used as a measure to lose weight or control any part of your life, but as a part of your self-care routine. Practicing gentle nutrition is mostly possible if you have a positive relationship with food, otherwise, your self-care routine may spin out of control, so it's important to work on your mindset first before implementing gentle nutrition in your life. Gentle nutrition's purpose is to nourish your body and mind in a non-restricted way where you practice unconditional love towards yourself.

Honoring your health starts from the inside. People that live healthy, unrestricted lifestyles know that health from the inside translates to health on the outside.

Chapter 2: Diets and Mentality

Do you eat to live or live to eat? This is an old saying implying that if you live to eat, you are leading an unhealthy lifestyle. That's debatable, though. In today's culture, someone who "lives to eat" can also be described as a foodie, and being a foodie doesn't require that you have to be addicted to food. Loving food can be a freeing experience, and you can still be an intuitive eater while being a foodie. What you can't be while you're a foodie is on a diet. The main difference between diet culture and intuitive eating is that one frees your mind and body, and the other places shackles on your mind and body, especially if you enjoy eating. Diet culture has been around for a long time, but as our food choices and options have become more and more unhealthy, and the culture of eating more and more prevalent in societal and social activities, diet culture has tried to adapt by becoming more and more extreme. Diet culture is literally everywhere, and it has become quite the industry. If you were to gain a few pounds during the winter and find that the denim cutoffs you bought last summer don't want to go all the way up, which one of the gazillion diets are you going to use to lose the weight? Stop right there and first find out what diets and obsessive eating are doing to your mind (Korodetz, 2017).

What Diet Culture Does to Your Mind

To be the most healthy physically and mentally, you need to have a positive relationship with food. The first thing dieting does is takes away the positive association you have with food by telling you that there are foods that you can't eat, that some foods are bad for you, and that taking weight-loss supplements and shakes is a better option than nourishing yourself the traditional, age-old way. It is important to realize that diet culture is a highly profitable industry, and the industry's goal is to try and convince you that you need to make certain restrictions to your diet, purchase "weight-loss enhancing" products, and follow trends. When you go onto Instagram or YouTube, there is a plethora of content creators, each telling you to eat differently, cook your food in a different way, cut out different foods, and use certain products when you are dieting. Are these individuals really there to help you, or to keep you coming back to watch their next post?

When you are caught up in the diet culture, you may decide to follow "Slim Sindy" on Instagram because she recently lost 10 lbs on her new apple water cleanse. But here's the trap that's waiting for you after your last day of consuming Slim Sindy's disgusting apple water: if you don't continue doing the cleanse on some type of routine basis, those pounds, which were most likely water-weight, are going to come right back, possibly bringing along some of their friends, and this will affect your self-esteem, confidence, and belief in your own abilities. Diet culture is toxic for the mind and even more so for the body. Can you imagine anything more confusing for your body than yo-yo dieting?

One of the problems with nutrition and dieting is that we want to see results quickly. We live in an insta-world where everything is readily available, and we expect the same from whatever diet we decide to follow. These expectations can lead to disorderly thoughts and behaviors related to food and eating. Diet culture puts so much pressure on us to look a certain way that we feel like we'll do anything to achieve this. This pressure leads to the development of disordered eating. Disordered eating is the opposite of intuitive eating; in disordered eating, instead of eating based on what your body tells you and your intuition, your eating habits are based on external factors like societal norms. When you allow societal trends to tell you what and how much to eat, you are prone to developing disorderly eating, which is characterized by a period of restrictive eating as prescribed by society, which is then countered by a complete rebellious reaction to it, which is a binge episode. Many dietitians and professionals refer to this pattern as the "dieting pendulum," as it swings from one extreme to the other. After a binge, you will most likely have intense feelings of guilt and shame and start another restrictive eating period, and the rest is history. Although at this stage, the eating pattern is labeled as disordered, the individual displaying this behavior does not have an eating disorder. If the condition is not treated, however, it can develop into a serious condition like Anorexia, or Bulimia Nervosa, where the individual will eventually start purging after excessive eating episodes (Andrea Hardy, 2019).

An important question is whether some individuals are more prone to conform to the toxic diet culture than others. The answer to this is yes. Individuals who have insecurities or who suffer from low self-esteem are more likely to embrace the damaging and toxic effects of the diet culture in an attempt to improve themselves from society's perspective. As we said earlier, if you have a good relationship with food, it is good for your physical and mental health. If you are motivated to do extreme calorie-cutting, exercise too much or too hard, take pills or shakes, or do extreme restrictions, then you are in the web of the toxic diet culture. Usually someone decides to take this route because they see themselves, especially their body, as flawed and there is something about themselves that they want to change. However, even after they've reached their goal, they are not always satisfied, and sometimes, they are not even able to see the results for what they are—drastic. If someone like this is not able to see changes in their body even though there are changes, the issue is mental, and their starting point should not be food or exercise, but on a mental approach and possibly therapy. Being mentally healthy is extremely important if you want to make intuitive eating part of your life, so in the next chapter, we're going to focus on mindfulness and how to realize how awesome you really are (Compton, 2020).

Remember that diet culture exists because of these unnecessary insecurities; we keep diet culture alive by purchasing the products that its ambassadors claim will make us 'acceptable' to society. Society who? Become your own person, define your own society, and find the peace you are yearning for.

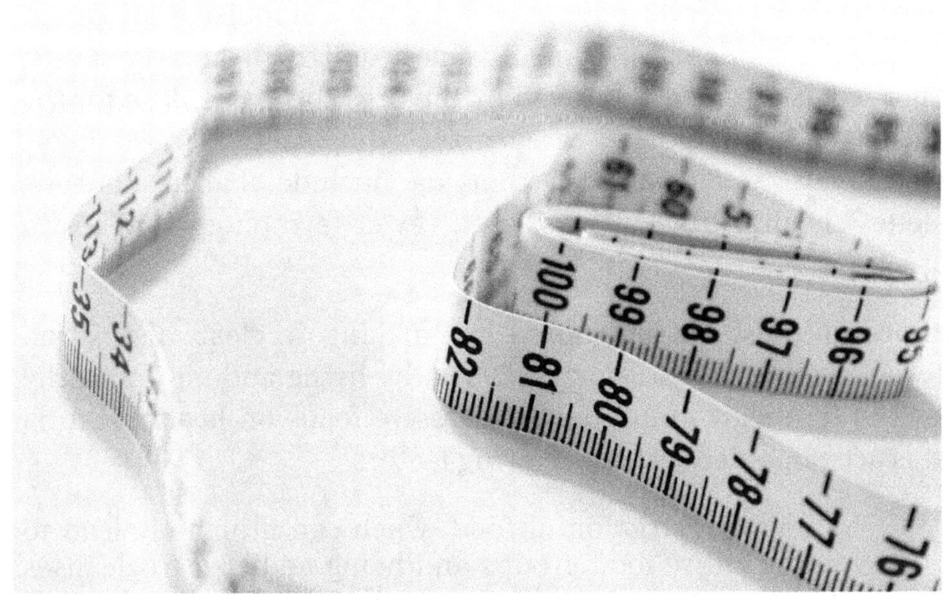

Orthorexia Nervosa

Most of us have heard of Anorexia and Bulimia Nervosa, and we know that these are serious eating disorders, but what is Orthorexia Nervosa? Those with this condition are concerned with healthy eating, so it can't possibly be that bad. However, according to medical experts, Orthorexia can become just as serious as Anorexia and Bulimia Nervosa. It is a fixation on healthy eating and a healthy lifestyle, wherein the individual becomes so obsessive that they develop an eating disorder based on the extreme health craze and diet culture we are currently experiencing. Orthorexia, if left untreated, can have severe consequences. The orthorexic's obsession is linked to food quality and not quantity, as is the case with other eating disorders, so individuals with orthorexia are not that focused on losing weight. However, one common denominator that has appeared during recent studies is that individuals who have this eating disorder are prone to have conditions like obsessive-compulsive disorder, perfectionist tendencies, control issues, and high anxiety levels. Orthorexia is often partly driven by the urge to stay healthy for the sake of an individual's career, accordingly, the most likely professionals to develop Orthorexia include ballet dancers, athletes, healthcare workers, and even symphony orchestra musicians.

Orthorexia must be diagnosed by making a clear distinction between a normal obsession with healthy living and an unhealthy one. The first sign would be an obsessive focus on healthy eating that is accompanied by the following factors:

1. The severe restriction of food which can ultimately lead to avoiding entire food groups and being addicted to cleanses and prolonged fasting. There should also be an indication that this behavior is becoming more severe as time goes on.
2. When any rules are broken that this individual has imposed on themselves, they experience extreme anxiety that can manifest physically.
3. They are constantly preoccupied with what the best dietary choices are to promote their physical health.

Another giveaway is that these behaviors make it impossible for them to go through the daily motions because of their compulsive nature. These compulsive behaviors can be disruptive in several different ways:

1. They can experience health issues due to food restrictions that led to serious and debilitating health conditions.
2. Due to anxiety and compulsive behavior, they find it difficult to navigate normal social situations.

3. These individuals are also usually emotionally dependent and are excessively focused on body image, their identity, and their self-worth.

The negative effects one can suffer from when they have Orthorexia are severe and can both be physical and mental. This is what happens when you get caught in the web of diet culture and get a distorted idea of what health is and what it should be. Always make sure that you have a balanced sense of self and understanding of food. One of the best ways to develop this mindset is through intuitive eating (Petre, 2020).

Principle 2: Reject the Diet Mentality

Of course, intuitive eating will reject the toxic diet mentality, and that is why it is one of the ten principles that underlie intuitive eating. If you have been hooked on fad diets all your life, this may not be an easy process for you to engage with, and surprisingly enough, the place to start is not going to be your eating habits. In order to reject diet culture and the diet mentality, one needs to do some introspection to see if there are any insecurities or unresolved psychological issues that need attention.

Think about what and who you're following on social media. Do you follow any diet or fitness influencers? Are they certified nutritionists or are they just girls who say they eat specific things but actually, you have no idea what they really eat because you only watch their videos that they shoot at a specific time and edit with a certain idea in mind?

We can also make these videos and portray our lives in a certain way. Except for the fact that we have other jobs, other responsibilities, and other things we need to do. It's important to understand that appearance is not everything as it is portrayed in advertising, the media, and social media. But it's hard because it is literally all around us. Let's move on to focus on self-love and how it can help us to cultivate healthier intuitive eating habits.

Chapter 3: The Perfection in Imperfection

Intuitive eating is the whole package, which means it's meant for life. Once you start adopting its mindful practices to improve yourself, the effects will cause a ripple of health and happiness that stretches into a space of permanency. However, because it is the whole package, it requires you to work on more than just your eating habits. One of the things that give the soul freedom and happiness is self-love, and one of the ways to show yourself that you are important is by practicing self-care. The pursuit of perfection has gotten more prominent in our lives since the dawn of the internet and social media. How do we decide what's perfect and what's not? And who gets to decide whether you're perfect or imperfect? The truth is that nothing is perfect, which means everything is imperfect. And if everything is imperfect, you can just as well see imperfection as a form of perfection and embrace it. As Leonard Cohen famously said, "there's a crack in everything; that's how the light gets in" (McGinley, 2017).

Embracing Imperfection in Yourself

If you don't know how to make that mind shift and start seeing the beauty in yourself, it's time to loosen up a little and start doing things that make you forget of being consciously aware of your 'imperfections.'

First, take your gaze from yourself and focus it on others. Look for what you would call 'imperfections.' What do you see? And, more importantly, how do you react to what you see? When you look at someone else, do you notice their beauty first or their imperfections or flaws? People who are very insecure would try to identify a flaw first, while people who are more comfortable with themselves may not even pay so much attention to how someone else looks. The same goes for you—the way you look at other people and what you notice about them first says a lot about how you see yourself.

When you go into the bathroom in the morning to brush your teeth and you look in the mirror, do you want to see a flaw? Do you have a 'favorite' flaw that you like to focus on if other flaws, like a new zit, are not noticeable on that particular day? (No zits today, let's move back to my big nose.) I think most of us have experienced this feeling! What you need is a pack of sticky notes and a black marker to put beside your bathroom ksin. Try this experiment for a week. Each time you walk into the bathroom and look into the mirror, write down the first thought that comes up into your head in big, thick letters and stick it up against the wall or the top part of the mirror. No cheating! Was it positive, negative, or neutral? At the end of the week, collect all the sticky notes from your wall. There's probably going to be quite a few, as you may use the mirror more than once a day. These sticky notes will reflect your level of self-love and tell you which parts of yourself you need to embrace and start showing some love and appreciation! For the next week (make sure you have enough sticky notes), you need to have your sticky notes ready every time you approach the mirror in your bathroom. This week is when you'll start embracing your imperfections by using positive affirmations. When you look in the mirror and you experience a positive thought, write it down, and stick your victory post on the wall or mirror. If it's more to the negative side, write a counter-approach. For example, if you observe something in the mirror that you don't like, instead of writing why you don't like it, take note of why it is a valuable part of your life and makes you who you are. Then, stick it next to all of your other stickies, and have a reflection session at the end of the week. Was there a drastic change in your perception or only a small one? Did you manage to identify the positive in what you see as an imperfect feature? Even the smallest changes in how you approached seeing yourself is a victory, and if the sticky notes work for you, try doing it for a few more weeks. Otherwise, you can start practicing these positive affirmations in your head every time you see yourself and feel negativity creeping up.

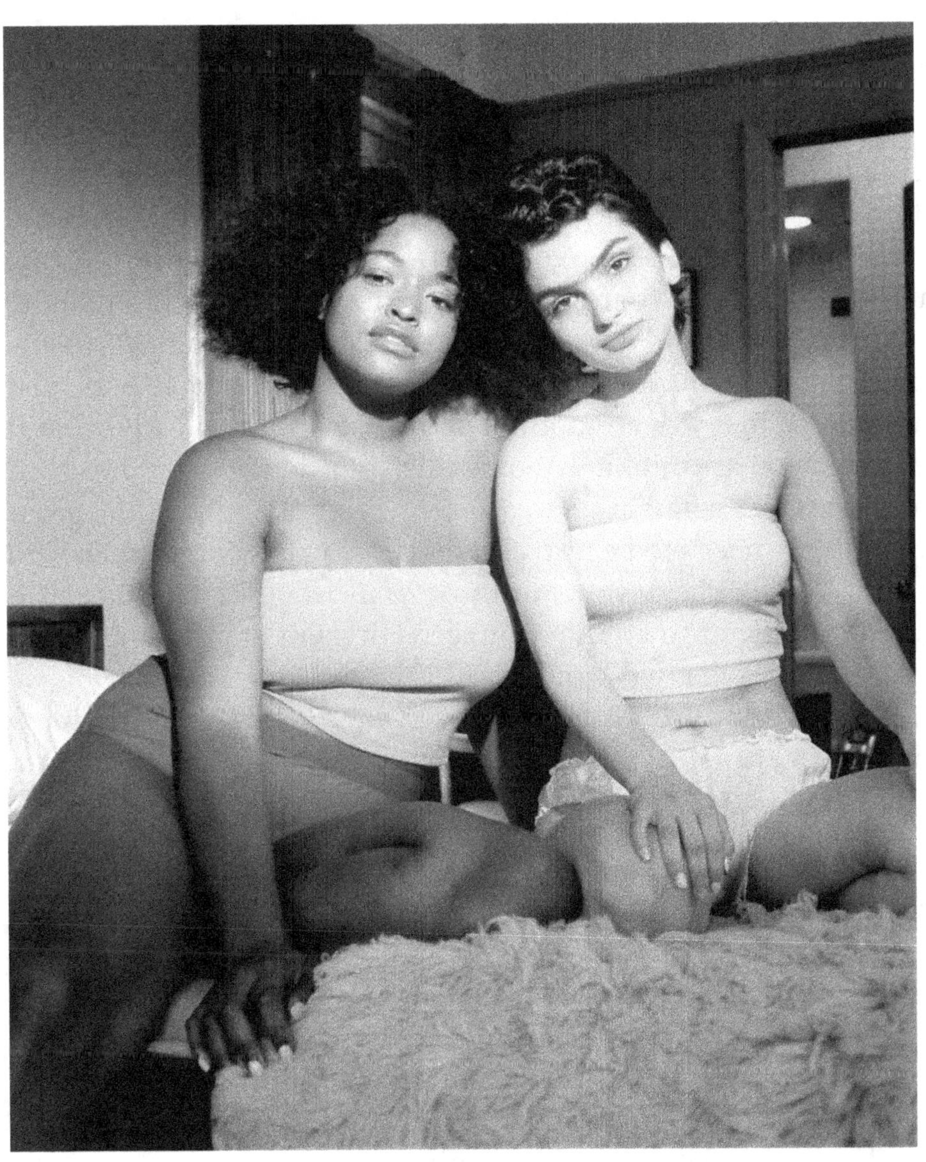

Embracing Imperfections in Your Circumstances

One of the things diet culture teaches us is that we need to perfect our habits and that there is little room for spontaneity or unforeseen circumstances that can cause us to eat that dreaded donut. This mindset is not going to free you or make you feel that you are in charge of your body or your life. Ironically, it's going to do the opposite, and you are going to feel like you are losing control. The reason for this is because by following a specific diet or eating regime, you are not necessarily giving your body what it needs, and you are definitely not giving your mind what it needs. It is also true that some of us thrive on structure and need it in our lives, but this needs to be a structure that you are comfortable with and that doesn't choke you. For those of us who like structure, it is also more difficult to embrace imperfections in our circumstances because it feels like we are being thrown off track. And when we feel like we're thrown off track, at least in my experience, it's easy to just give up instead of seeing the imperfection for what it is, a minor detour, and getting back on the main road in your life.

Freedom is accepting the imperfect. Freedom is in approaching imperfect circumstances with open arms and finding solutions. Finally, freedom is in positivity and proactively looking at how you can swerve past these obstacles if you know they are on your road ahead. That being said, if encountering them is inevitable, go with it, and enjoy the ride. Tensing up and freaking out is likely going to lead to you picking up the pieces later. Just remember to breathe. Take the good and leave the bad behind.

Principle 3: Cope With Your Emotions Using Kindness

Emotional eating is when we eat for reasons that have little to do with physical hunger. If you realize that you are emotionally eating, your first reaction may be to be critical towards yourself. Kindness is what you need at this point, because there's a reason you are doing this. Emotional eating is often a coping mechanism, and while there is nothing wrong with eating to celebrate an event or eating good food because you like food, emotional eating often goes with overeating. A functional approach is to observe what triggers you to start an emotional eating episode and to try and identify the underlying factors. For example, is it an emotional trigger or can it possibly be stress? Dealing with the underlying issue by being kind to yourself can help you free yourself from emotional eating, which can also be a form of restriction in your life. If you feel you need to talk to someone and spill the beans in confidentiality, that can also help a lot.

Chapter 4: What is Hunger?

One of the big debates about emotional eating is how to deal with hunger, how to understand hunger, and what it means to embrace hunger. One of the biggest critiques diet culture has of the intuitive eating approach is that it encourages people to eat more and doesn't necessarily teach them important information about macros, calorie-counting, portion size, and so on. A great way to start this discussion is by looking at the science behind hunger, and it is actually really helpful to understand the way your body can develop a habit of telling you you're hungry when you're actually not. Before I say too much, let's look at what the science says.

The Science Behind Hunger

Most of us are taught that, if we experience that pang of hunger, it is a sign that our body needs nourishment. But can your brain be fooling you into thinking you need food when you don't? It all comes down to where that signal comes from and how it is regulated.

When your body is giving you those hunger signals, this can be either two types of hunger—homeostatic hunger or hedonic hunger. There's a big difference between these two types of hunger, and knowing the difference and which one signals real hunger can make you a healthier individual. Homeostatic hunger is when your body is low on energy and is telling you that you need to fuel up. When you are low on energy, your brain secretes the hormone 'ghrelin,' which is also known as the "hunger hormone" to remind you to eat something. As soon as you start eating something, your brain suppresses this signal. On the other hand, there is hedonistic hunger, which is closely linked with our love for eating tasty food. You can experience hedonic hunger even if your body isn't low on energy. For example, after having lunch, you may be walking by a bakery, see the most delectable cupcake, and buy and eat it just because it's so yummy. That's how hedonistic hunger works. Most junk food contains preservatives like MSG which makes you crave those snacks even more after you've consumed loads of them, which completely confuses your body. You know what I mean, eating that extra slice of pizza because pepperoni garlic is your favorite kind and you just want one more little piece. In these cases, hedonistic hunger can mess with your health and your weight if you are not tuned in to what your body needs and when it has received enough food. Ultimately, you are playing a confusing game with your brain, which needs to secrete the right hormones to keep you healthy (Miller, 2016).

This doesn't mean that homeostatic hunger only permits you to eat certain foods or to never indulge in things you enjoy, it's simply that if you know your body and you are tuned into your hunger signals, you'll know when to say yes, when to say no, when to eat a whole donut, and when to just take a bite to savor the taste because that's all your body has space for.

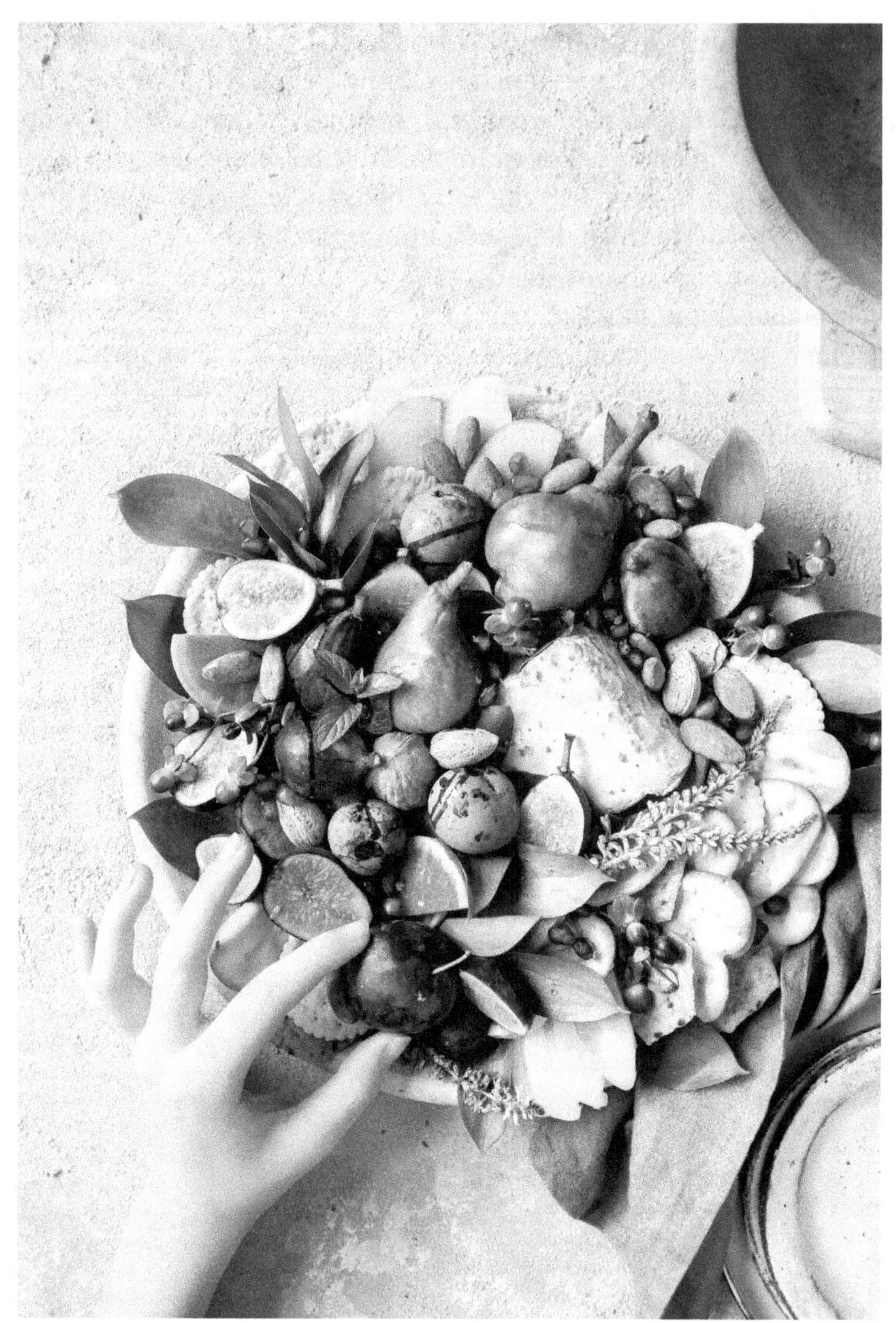

How In Tune Are You With Your Hunger?

Let's sketch three scenarios, each one a bit different from the one before. Read each one while considering your normal eating behavior, and decide which one describes you best. Then, read the interpretation of each to see how differently hunger can be approached and how it can affect one's health and happiness.

Scenario 1

You're invited to dinner with friends. You were a bit hungry a few hours before, so you had half of a sandwich. When you arrive, you see that your friends have prepared this massive spread that contains some of your favorite foods. Even though you're a little bit full, you dish up like there's no tomorrow and you clear your plate. Then, they also bring dessert even though you're really stuffed. Who says no to dessert? You dish yourself a generous portion and finish it even though you were already semi-full when you arrived and stuffed after you finished dinner. Feeling like a pufferfish, you take your last sip of wine and go home.

Scenario 2

You're invited to dinner with friends. You were a bit hungry before dinner, but you decided to save yourself for your friend's famous homemade pizza. You arrive at your friend's house absolutely ravenous and eat four massive deep dish squares of freshly-baked goodness in record time. Afterward, you knew you actually had enough after the second slice, but it was just too good and you were starving! When you are offered dessert, you politely decline but feel a bit bummed out because you wanted to taste your friend's homemade chocolate fondant. On the way home, you make a pact with yourself to try and control yourself while you're eating.

Scenario 3

You're invited to dinner with friends. You feel a bit hungry beforehand, but you know your friend is going to go all out, so you just eat a handful of berries to fill you up temporarily. You arrive at your friend's house not starving but not full, and you enjoy a piece of pizza. You want another piece because it's really good, but you feel satisfied, so you say no. For dessert, you get your own little chocolate fondant in a ramekin. It smells delicious. You take a few bites until you feel the sweetness becomes too much, and you put your spoon down. Feeling light and refreshed, yet nourished and full, you say goodbye to your friends and are on your way home.

Did any of these scenarios resonate with you? More than one resonated with me as I think back to my own journey that led to intuitive eating. Here's the reveal. Go to the scenario you identified with the most, and read it first. Then, read ahead to see how those scenarios relate to the behavior described in each case.

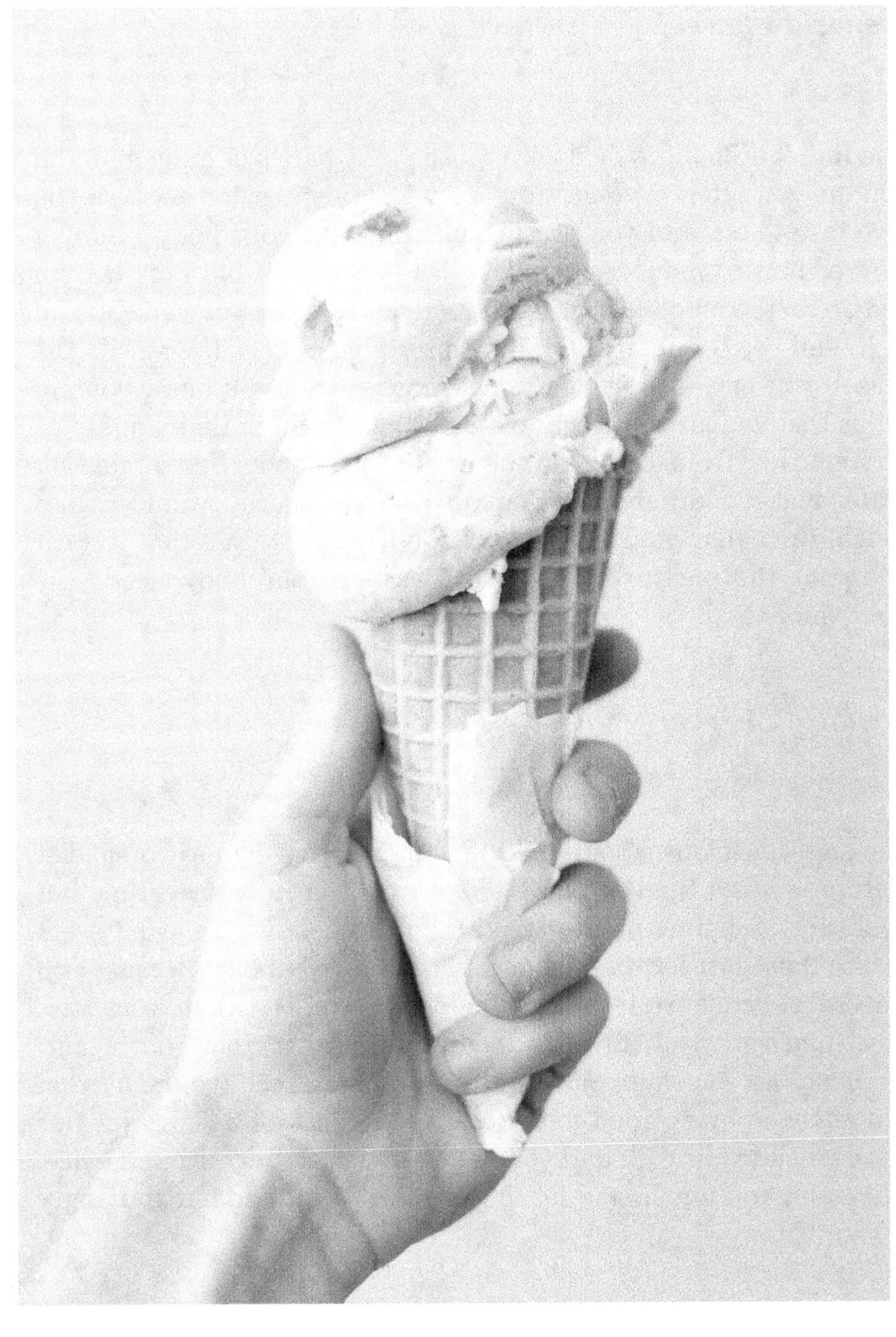

Scenario 1 Reveal

You find it difficult to deal with those pesky pangs of hunger, and if you do, you often overeat. You are a hedonistic eater because you love tasty food, and you are not in tune with your body's hunger cues or how to manage them. You will also eat something tasty if you are in the mood for eating. If food tastes good, you can eat a lot of it, and you'll only feel the uncomfortable effects afterward. The reason you may also decide to eat more even if you know you are full is that you are an emotional eater or you think that you are so far removed from being in tune with your body that it doesn't really make a difference. You do not necessarily want to lose weight or change your eating habits, but they indicate that you eat more for the pleasure of it than because your body needs the nourishment.

Scenario 2 Reveal

You are conscious about dieting, but you have more of a diet culture mindset than listening to your body. You enjoy eating, but you want to maintain your weight, and somehow, you can't seem to lose those last few pesky pounds around your belly. Because you starved yourself, you couldn't help but overeat when you were presented with your favorite food, and you had that "not again" moment, as this happens quite often. You keep yourself from genuinely enjoying good food because of a lack of balance in your mindset and your diet, and you ended up restricting yourself twice, still eating too much, and leaving the party guilt-ridden and angry at yourself.

Scenario 3 Reveal

When you felt hungry before going to dinner at your friend's, you knew that eating something heavy like a sandwich would make you lose your appetite, so you literally shushed the loudest hunger pang with a handful of berries. When eating the pizza, you were able to enjoy the flavor and because you were not ravenous, you could focus on the conversation around you and eat slowly. This is why you needed less food to feel satisfied. After the pizza, you could feel that you were quite full, so you just took a bite or two from the fondant to get a taste of the sweet treat. You left feeling light as a feather and physically and mentally satisfied.

Which one are you, which one do you think is the best for your body and mind, and which one do you want to be? In the next chapter, we'll be looking at how to develop an intuitive eating mindset.

Principle 4: Feel Your Fullness

This principle is relevant to the concept of homeostatic hunger. What it means is that if you feel that first signal of fullness, that's when you've had enough. If your eating habits have been based on hedonistic hunger for a long time, you may not be able to experience that initial feeling of satiety anymore, as your body is conditioned to eat more than is required. In this case, you need to train your body to be able to feel its natural impulses again because it's important to honor your body's signals of fullness for the sake of your health and not to keep on eating for other reasons. Everyone's body is different, therefore portion sizes are just a general guideline. It's important to listen to your body and know that your body most likely requires less food than what you are currently consuming. Social eating is part of our culture, and that is one of the reasons we tend to eat more. Honor your body—feel your fullness.

Chapter 5: "Get" Yourself to Get the Mindset

The intuitive eating mindset is not only a positive mindset towards food but also towards yourself and your body image. If you have been on an emotional eating journey for some time or you just enjoy eating and you often overeat, then you need to relearn the cues and signals your body sends you and to trust your body.

"Getting" Yourself

We are all different types of eaters, just as we are all individuals. We have different favorite foods, we like different flavors and smells, and some of us are salty and some are sweet. So, what does this have to do with developing an intuitive eating mindset? First, if you are not in tune with your body at the moment, it's important to understand yourself so you can figure out why this is happening and what you can do to change that. So many of us are too hard on ourselves because we are looking for a (stereo)type of what we see as perfection, not realizing that we are perfection. So, here is your "getting yourself" toolkit that you can use to develop the healthiest version of yourself you can possibly be:

- Are you overcritical of yourself? Do you often have negative thoughts about yourself? If so, this can be one of your biggest obstacles if you want to experience the freedom of intuitive eating because you are holding yourself back. Many of us are perfectionists by nature, and this automatically tends to make us more self-critical, especially if we cannot master a new skill quickly or get something as perfectly as we see it in our minds. If you think about it this way, is it possible that one of those things you can't seem to "get right" might be your body? Did someone tell you that you need to fix your body? Some women become self-critical due to the idea of perfection they see in the media, and others develop a distorted view of their bodies due to unfair criticism from their family or peers. This idea goes back to seeing perfection in imperfection. Was anyone who has ever criticized you absolutely flawless themselves? Do you think any picture or video you see in the media of an influencer or a celebrity has not been airbrushed, edited, or photoshopped? It's time to stop being your biggest enemy and let that hair down!

- Pep talk over—let's get down to business. To "get" yourself, you need to find the root of what's causing you to be your own enemy. Is being your own enemy what's keeping you going? Are you afraid to let go and just accept yourself? Why don't you do the following exercise to take the first step into really "getting" you:
    1. Grab a pen and a notepad.
    2. Make sure you're alone and that you are in a comfortable and pleasant environment where you can think clearly without interruption.
    3. Now, start thinking clearly and without interruption, and then write the following down:
        - 3 things about yourself that bother you the most.
        - Why you think these things bother you. If there's more than one reason, write down each one you think is relevant.
    4. Now, look at the reasons or causes you wrote down that explain why certain aspects of yourself bother you. Are any of these reasons still relevant to your life today? Or are you just still stuck with the effects they caused, meaning they are holding you back in life for no good reason?

If the reason you feel the way you feel about yourself is because of things that happened in the past, there is no reason for you to hold on to these feelings. If you're afraid to let those feelings go because you don't know what the next step in your life will be, don't be afraid, because the next step is to free your mind and your body and become a healthier and happier you. If you want something new to throw all your energy into after you've left the negativity behind, let it be your health and expanding your creativity and sense of self-worth.

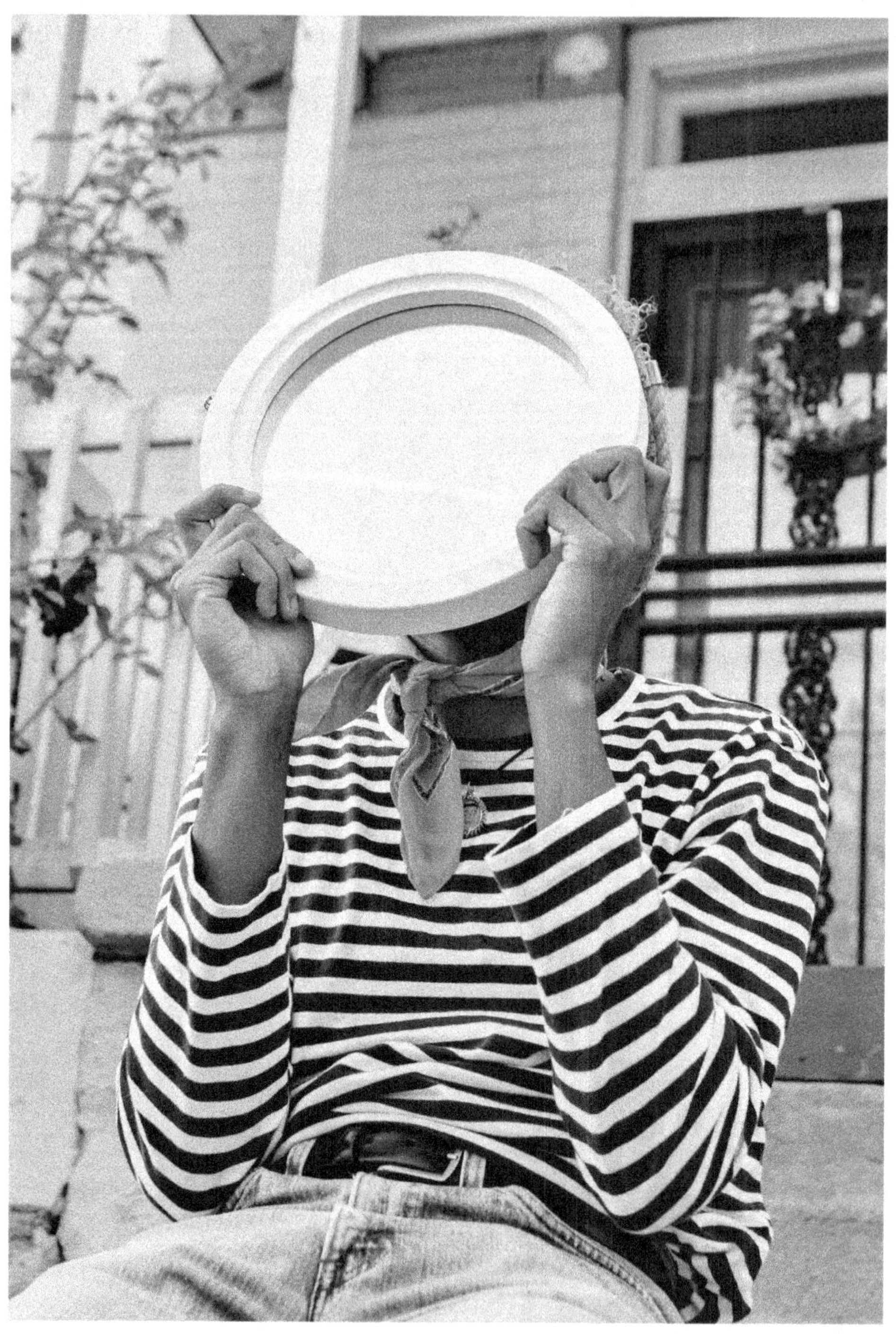

Getting the Mindset

Here are a few tips to start getting connected to your body again and to relearn that important intuition:

- Set an alarm for every few hours and spend a few minutes checking in with your body. Not hunger specifically, but with how you are feeling overall. For example, are you feeling calm, do you need to go to the restroom, and have you been thinking about work? Ruminate over everything you think about when the alarm goes off, and then wait for the next alarm before you do it again.
- Set a few rules for when you're eating. For example, remove all distractions around you. Put your phone in another room, turn off any music or anything you're watching so you can focus on eating mindfully. Take the time to taste your food and never try to eat in a whole meal when you are pressed for time. After each bite, listen to your body. You may find that you are satisfied much more quickly than usual.
- Is this pasta still tasting as good as I did when I took the first bite? If not, it's a sign that your satiety levels are going up and you may be full. Are you eating it just to clear your plate, or are you starting to feel a bit sluggish?
- Don't confuse the diet mentality with intuitive eating when it comes to food preparation—nobody wants to force limp, steamed vegetables with no flavor down their throats just because they have to. How do you like your broccoli? Sauteed in some butter and garlic? Do it. Intuitive eating is not about swallowing food without chewing just because it's low in calories.
- Have you ever spent an hour or two cooking a dish and then when the time comes to eat, you find that the sensory experience of cooking has taken away your appetite? This is an important part of intuitive eating—to make eating and cooking a sensory experience that you find pleasurable and enticing. Let all your senses be captivated by the food you eat. This is one of the reasons why limp broccoli won't work.

Experiment with flavors, make the cooking process a journey, and enjoy every moment that comes before eating.

- Nutrition is always important, but don't let it squash you back into the diet culture mold. For an intuitive eater, a productive approach toward healthier eating is to look at which nutritious foods you can add to your lifestyle instead of which foods you need to avoid. These foods will give your body the nutrients it needs, and this may subsequently cause you to crave less unhealthy food. The goal is to never focus on restriction but on food freedom (Holbrook, 2020).

Principle 5: Respect Your Body

Respecting your body begins with knowing and understanding your body and, most importantly, appreciating your body. This principle includes the concept of self-care and also showing compassion and patience instead of forcing your body into a mold. Respecting your body is linked to respecting your mind and yourself as an individual, and therefore having a positive outlook on yourself as well as life. This is an integral part of the intuitive eating approach. Shifting your focus away from what you perceive as physical imperfections toward everything your body is capable of doing for you is a productive way to gain respect for your body and to start treating it the way it deserves to be treated.

Chapter 6: The Food Police

Who's the food police? In most cases, it's ourselves, but when you become an intuitive eater or change your eating habits, the people around you can also start policing your eating habits. This is because of a strange phenomenon that exists in most of our lives—there are relationships in our lives we have with others that are kind of based on food and eating only. It can be the same with alcohol. You may have that friend that you only meet up with for cocktails, and the whole night is based around drinking, although not necessarily based on getting drunk. However, you don't really have anything else in common. So, when you meet up again and you don't feel like drinking alcohol and order a mocktail instead, what do you think your friend is going to say? If the act of drinking alcohol together is part of what cements the relationship, they are going to ask you questions because they don't want to feel left out or like the only one going wild while you sit there sipping your Virgin Margarita. It's the same with food, and strangely enough, married couples sometimes discover what a crucial role food plays in their relationship when one partner decides to change their lifestyle and the other is left behind, causing relationship problems. Let's go through all the possible food policemen in your life and how to handle them so intuitive eating doesn't make you feel guilty.

When You Are the Food Police

This is an internal matter that should be dealt with by looking at the reasons why you are policing yourself. There can be numerous possibilities. For example, you may be trying to be more intuitive when it comes to your eating habits, which is a good thing, but instead of being kind to yourself, you insert a nasty wedge of negativity between you and your goal of physical and mental freedom and wellbeing. If you're going to try to police yourself constantly, you're going to get the idea that you are more dependent on food than you really are because you are constantly thinking about food or giving food too much thought when you are confronted by it. One of the first things one realizes when intuitiveness "clicks" is that you have total freedom to eat what you like, but you really don't have that burning desire to eat everything you encounter because your body doesn't feel the need to eat as much. Thus, if you find that you are your own food police, this ties in with your perception about diet culture, and may be one way you are still allowing diet culture in your life without you realizing it. If the policing is happening, you're not experiencing the food freedom that you deserve, even if you are more in tune with your body. Letting go from the restrictions you set yourself and trusting your body is also important.

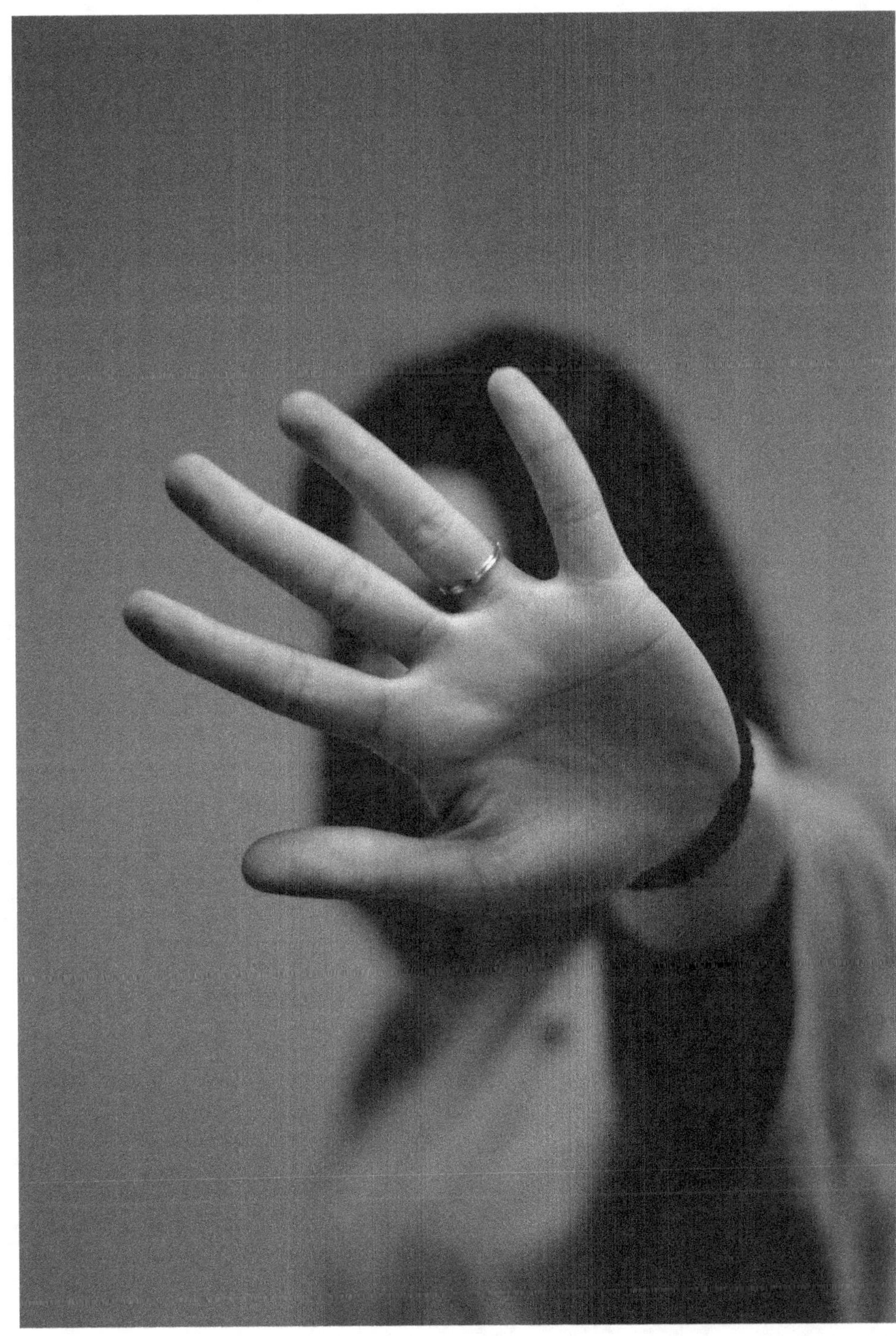

When Your Parents or Family Are Your Food Police

Due to the fact that diet culture, although not so extreme in the past, has existed for decades, many of us are and were policed as children by our parents, specifically our mothers, on what we eat, when we eat, and how much we eat. And, for many of us, that's where our issues with food come from—from our parents' issues with food. For example, imagine sitting at the dinner table and attempting to serve yourself another helping of mashed potatoes while getting the evil eye from your mother who is eating only a single pea for dinner. A growing child needs more calories and nourishment than an adult, so if a parent teaches their children healthy eating habits but then still polices what they eat, they are sabotaging their mission to raise healthy children. This may or may not be a description of your parents, but many individuals grow up confused about what they are actually supposed to do when a plate of food is put in front of them. And, of course, you don't want to upset your parents or make them angry. The answer is simple: eat what your body has space for and leave the rest. If you want another piece of chicken, then ignore the stiff atmosphere around the table and enjoy it. If the atmosphere is just too negative, have a snack at home, or consider talking to your parents about the food policing issue. Being an intuitive eater means you're going to be different from everyone else, even from other intuitive eaters, because our bodies have different needs. Your body comes first.

When Your Friends Are the Food Police

Do you have friends that police whether you eat, don't eat, or what you eat? This discussion can go in several directions because there may be several reasons why your friends are doing this. For example, friends can be competitive. If you go out to lunch with a friend and they want to order a burger but you want a chicken salad, this can upset them. Why aren't you also eating a burger with lots of bacon, cheese, and relish? Why are you trying to make them look like a gluttonous fatso while you plan on daintily picking at your salad? This really goes on in some people's minds because they are inherently competitive, and who is the best candidate for competition? Their best friend. Ironically, what they don't realize is that a restaurant chicken salad can also be loaded with calories, especially when it comes to the dressing, but the calorie component probably has nothing to do with why you ordered it if you are an intuitive eater. You just wanted a salad. And, if you eat your whole salad and they eat half their burger, you may very well have consumed more calories than they would have. The point is, they don't want to be the only one eating a burger, so they expect you to be a 'good friend' and eat one too. What this means is that they don't have the confidence to order what they want, so they are policing your choices to help them feel more supported in theirs.

Have you had this experience before? It is subtle competitiveness between friends that seems to be focused on eating and food. Sometimes the comment comes off as a joke, but behind that facade, there's no joke. You shouldn't have to choose between tuning in with your body or with your friends. Friends should respect each other's choices and own their own. If you want to order a triple-stacked burger with cheese sauce and extra bacon, then own it. If you only want to take two bites of that burger, then that's none of anyone's business, even if your friend finished a whole plate of fettuccine alfredo and a slice of cheesecake. Handling a situation like this may not be so easy as you are directly dealing with your friend's insecurities. Avoid becoming defensive, but stand your ground. Eat what your body needs, stop when it has had enough, and set an example for those around you.

Principle 6: Challenge the Food Police

We now know that the food police can manifest in many different ways, most commonly in our own heads due to external conditioning from diet culture and the overwhelming presence of social media. We have also established that the food police can be people around us and close to us—from our friends to our family. Remember to challenge the food police with kindness wherever you may encounter them. Food is not a good enough reason to damage your relationship with yourself, your family, or your friends. There is no shame in being healthy, and hopefully, your sense of enlightenment and contentment will rub off on those around you.

Chapter 7: The Food Pushers

Now that we know who the food police are, who are the food pushers? A food pusher is often associated with a motherly figure who is always cooking and gets great pleasure out of feeding those around her. It's their way to show love and affection, mixed with a strange approach to the traditional upbringing of being a good housewife. Quite often, food pushers also 'nourish' themselves with feeding, which is why they assume others would also feel loved by this gesture, but this is not always the case. How to deal with a food pusher if you're an intuitive eater is important, as there are usually no bad intentions behind them trying to stuff you with all kinds of baked and cooked goods; but you still have to find a way to politely decline.

How to Say No

"Why aren't you having some more?"

"Just a little bite; it won't hurt!"

"Loosen up and have a piece of pie with us!"

These are classic food pusher lines. The most common feeling you experience in this situation is guilt, which will make you eat something even if your body does not need the food and you may not feel hungry at all. Another difficult-to-navigate situation is a family gathering where social pressure can drive you to give in just to keep everyone happy.

"I made this especially for you because I know you like it!"

"It took aunt Jesse two hours to knead that dough, and you don't even want to taste a piece?"

"Are you feeling sick? Why are you eating so little?"

Hard times. The first thing you need to ask yourself is whose body is it? It's yours. Who is in charge of making decisions about the wellbeing of your body? You are. One strategy you can use is to politely decline when you are being offered food in a conniving way and then immediately change the subject. However, you need to be smart here. Changing the subject can seem obvious, so pick a topic that's going to captivate your audience. If it's the latest political or Hollywood gossip, go with it. If you don't have any idea what's happening in Hollywood, make something up. "Hey everyone, I heard that Nicholas Cage shaved off all his hair and went on a shoplifting rampage!" If you've got fact-checkers or Google addicts in the room, you may want to try another strategy, but this one usually works pretty well.

Another way of changing the subject without having the fact-checkers all over you is to start a conversation focusing on someone else in the room. "So, I heard that you and John are planning on buying a house! How many bedrooms, and are you looking in the suburbs?" That's a lot to answer, and it may redirect the entire conversation if you keep stoking the fire.

The food pusher may become so insistent that you may have to pull them aside and have a private conversation with them. Hopefully this doesn't happen, but as people have different personalities and some are more persistent and strong-willed than others, this is also a possibility. In this case, tell them that you've made some choices, that they have improved your life in several aspects, and that it has nothing to do with the food itself—you've always loved their food. They may possibly ask you if you are on a diet, in which case you can tell them no, because you are not. You can just tell them that you are relying more on your body to tell you when you need to eat instead of eating at scheduled times and eating specific quantities of food. Maybe, just maybe, they simply needed to understand (Comas, 2015).

How to Say No Version 2

Here are some other approaches you can consider that are also very useful when dealing with your friendly neighborhood food pusher:

- **Create a diversion:** This type of diversion is different than changing the topic of conversation. When you create a diversion, you are removing yourself from the situation so you can avoid the confrontational question. You can do this by saying you just remembered you need to ask your sister something important or that you need to quickly visit the restroom. If you are brave, you can throw in a little promise of taking a bite when you get back. If your food pusher has a memory of an elephant, like my grandmother used to have, they'll be sure to hold you accountable the moment you return.
- **Deflection:** This is a smart approach if you have a proper understanding of the food pusher's basic psychology and mindset. Often, food pushers offer those around them more food because they want more food but they don't want to eat alone. If this is the case, all you need to do is politely decline, compliment their food, and offer them more of their own food. Works like a charm.
- **Delay, delay, delay:** If it happens that you have some food on your plate and your food pusher is offering you more, use your remaining food as a weapon of delay by telling your host how much you are enjoying these last few bites and that you want to savor them before you consider having some more. The compliment will be well-received and there's no doubt that the food was tasty anyway. However, if you can't finish your plate, just use this delay

tactic and push the food around a little until dinnertime is over.

- **Keep a light atmosphere:** A little joke never hurt anyone. Joking or making a light humorous comment about how full you are and how eating another crumb would be spoiling the whole experience for you because it would just be one bite too much might diffuse the situation. This could work if your host has a light-hearted sense of humor.
- **Your final option:** Say no politely. No thank you. The only tricky part here is to say it in a way your host/food pusher will appreciate and understand. If you know them well, this shouldn't be a problem, except if you know they tend to be quite difficult, in which case one of the previous options may be more suitable. Your best bet is to just be sincere and genuine, which will be easy because that's most likely how you'll feel about the situation. If your food pusher strapped you to your chair and was literally trying to push a spoonful of peas down your esophagus before you had the chance to say no thank you, it would be understandable that sincerity may be difficult. Otherwise, being yourself and doing your best to appease your food pusher while politely declining can work for you (Xen and the Art of Mindful Eating, 2016).

To be honest, this chapter makes intuitive eating sounds like you're trying to hide something from your friends and family. This is not the case—what you are doing is adopting a healthy lifestyle that is still foreign to many people, and if they don't understand the principles behind intuitive eating and the physical and mental benefits that support it, they are likely to misinterpret your sometimes uncharacteristic behavior. They are also likely to feel excluded, offended, and a range of other emotions because intuitive eating is unconventional in the diet culture environment we live in, but it appears to make people healthier and happier while eating what they love. That can, understandably, be confusing. So, although all of these deflection methods may make you feel like a spy, they are there to help you cope with people you love but don't understand your lifestyle. People who are genuinely caring and loving are still human. Patience is key.

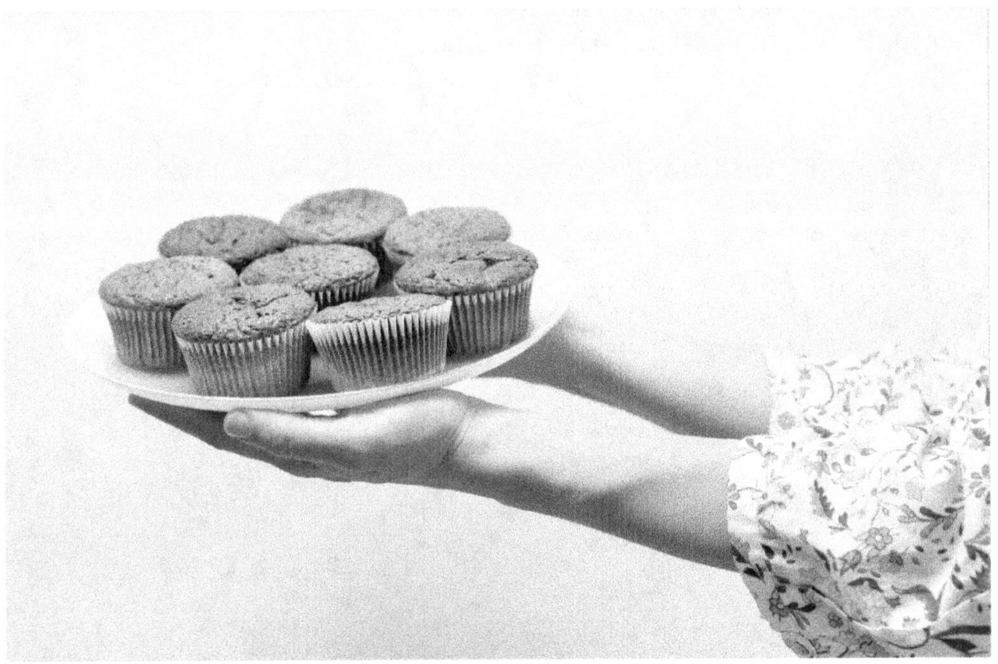

Principle 7: Discover the Satisfaction Factor

When you start to know your body and the way it communicates with you, you will also start to understand the difference between being full and being satisfied. Being satisfied is linked to filling a need other than just bodily hunger, while fullness means that your body has had enough to eat. This is one of the most challenging aspects of your journey towards intuitive eating, as intuitive eating only requires you to be full and seek satisfaction elsewhere because you know that eating more than you need does not provide healthy satisfaction. Doing something productive with your mind like meditation or acquiring a new skill can bring you healthy satisfaction. Cultivating and nurturing your relationships can bring you satisfaction. If you are not able to tell the difference yet, it is hard to know when your body has had enough food. This is part of your intuitive eating journey, and just starting off by being aware of the two concepts can help you focus on telling them apart and identifying them as two distinct feelings.

Chapter 8: Moving From Chronic Dieting to Intuitive Eating

The dieting industry is not only all around us, it is toxic because it sends a false message of attainability that leads its followers into a trap of yo-yo dieting, self-esteem issues, and even disordered eating. Removing your mind completely from that paradigm is tough, but deciding to take the first step and starting to change your mindset is a giant leap in the right direction. What makes intuitive eating different from any other diet is that the change starts in your mind and not by weighing ingredients, restricting your calories, or sticking to a certain exercise regime. It requires you to be brutally honest with yourself in order to cultivate that change to mental health. Another approach to eating, called mindful eating, can help you with the bulk of the mindset changes. Mindfulness can be defined as a type of meditative approach to life where you shift your focus and awareness to that which you are feeling in the moment without being judgmental about those feelings or applying any type of interpretation. Mindfulness is used to relax the body and mind and also to develop a more relaxed but focused approach to life in general (Mayo Clinic Staff, 2021). Mindfulness has also been applied to eating, and learning to approach eating in a mindful way first can help you change your mindset and approach to food and eating to be more healthy and focused towards what your body needs.

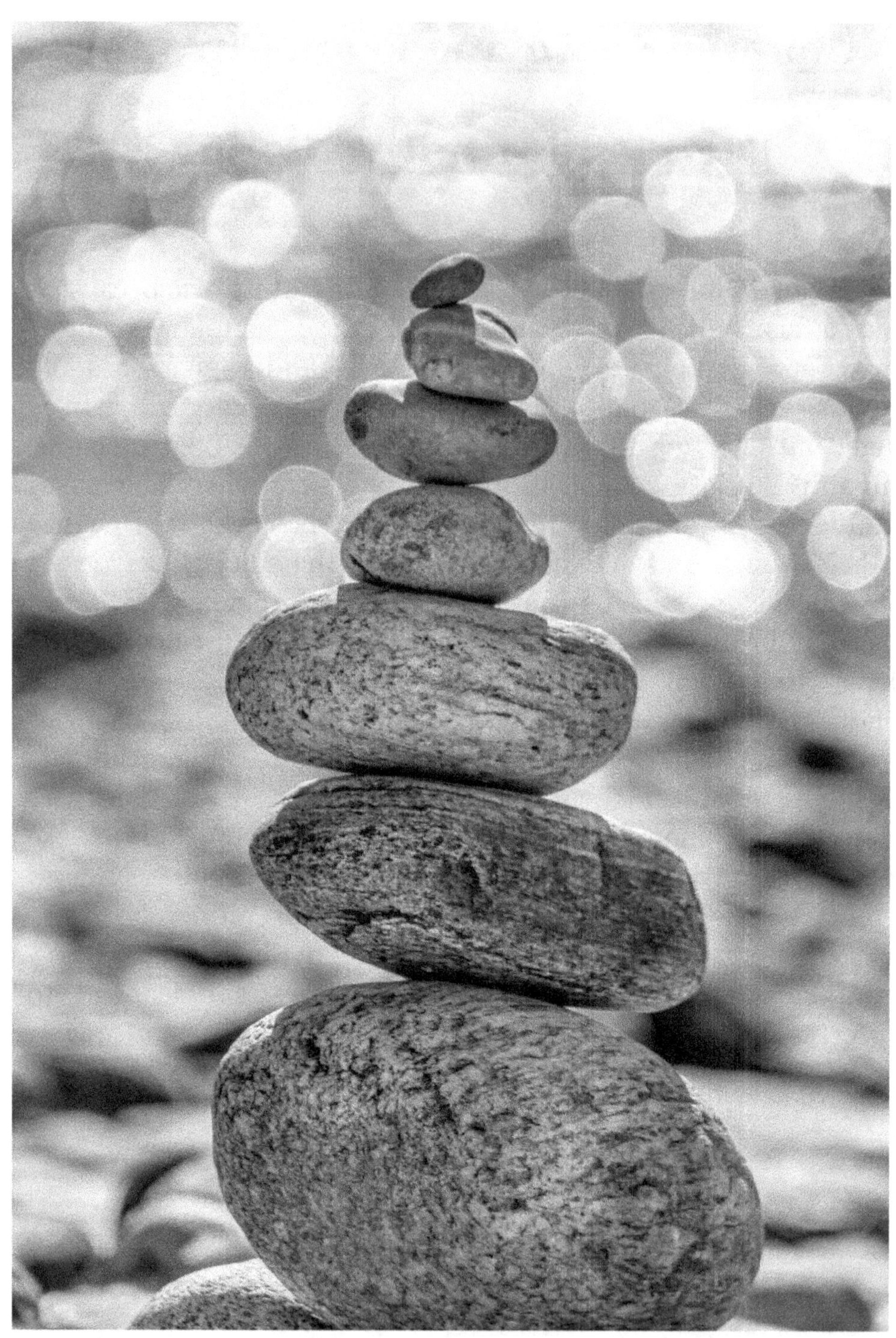

The Mindful Eating Stepping Stone

Mindful eating is a great tool to help you not only gain control over your eating habits, but also develop a relationship of understanding with food and stop unhealthy eating habits like bingeing or obsessive calorie counting. Mindful eating involves reaching a state where you can focus all of your attention on what you are experiencing and feeling while you are eating, your cravings, and any physical cues related to eating you may feel. Here is a summary of what mindful eating is based on:

- Paying attention to your physical hunger cues and then only consuming food until you get that indication of fullness.
- Practicing eating without any distractions and eating slowly.
- Appreciating and enjoying your food.
- Paying attention to the reaction your body and your feelings have from food.
- Focusing on eating for the purpose of overall wellbeing and health.
- Learning coping mechanisms that help you deal with food-related anxiety and guilt.
- Being able to tell the difference between real hunger and non-hunger-related prompts.
- Focusing on your senses when you are eating by smelling, looking, tasting, and feeling the textures of the food.

These fundamental elements of mindful eating promote a more conscious and thoughtful approach to eating instead of an impulse-based approach. Most of us have most likely practiced mindless eating at some point in our lives, where you just gobble up a sandwich for the sake of it. Maybe you do it every day because you need to eat but you don't think about what you eat or how much your body needs for satiety. One of the reasons mindless eating is unhealthy and, well, mindless, is because your brain takes up to 20 minutes before it sends you that "I'm full now, you can stop eating" signal. Here, I am referring to the genuine satiety signal and not the satisfaction signal as we discussed in the 7th principle of intuitive eating. What mindful eating will do is help you transition from the diet culture restrictive mindset to a freer mindset by helping you identify your triggers and tune you in to your body's cues (Bjarnadottir, 2019).

Our good friends at Harvard University have created a guide that will help you to ease into a mindful approach to eating. Following a guide to start eating with more freedom sounds counterintuitive, yes, but the purpose of the guide is to help you get rid of unhealthy habits. If you've been disconnected from your body for a long time, connecting again actually takes commitment and a belief in yourself; and having a guide as a backbone to fall back onto can serve as a support system for you to grow your wings and eventually fly with confidence. Although the mindful eating approach also involves opting for healthy food choices, what we need to focus on now is the approach and attitude toward food in general and not any diet-related or nutritionally restrictive approaches, as they are not relevant to intuitive eating. Consider the following points and contemplate whether you currently apply them to your approach to eating:

1. Start the mindful process when you go shopping for food. Whether you make a list or you like to go and look at what's available at your local grocery store, consider the quality and significance of each item you place into your shopping cart. How is this food going to benefit you and nourish you? Are you going to enjoy the food and can you cook it in a way you like? By following this consideration process, you avoid impulsively placing items in your shopping cart that can lead to mindless eating later on.
2. Make sure that you are never starving before eating a meal but eat when you are hungry. Starving yourself makes you eat too fast and too much, which leaves your stomach carrying an overload of food and not being able to tell you when it has reached its satiety level. Eating should be about nourishing your body, not about filling a void.

3. Give your stomach the benefit of the doubt by dishing up a small portion first. Your stomach is only the size of your fist and stuffing a loaded plate of food in there is actually hard to picture.
4. Learn to appreciate every bite and every chew. If you're eating something that grosses you out, then this is not going to work. But the point is to enjoy your food, so, in terms of this premise, let's assume that you're eating food you like. Make the most of the moment and feel how it gives strength back to your body. You can take a moment before you start your meal and observe your food, the effort that went into making it, and express gratitude for the privilege of being able to eat good food.
5. Make your meal a multisensory experience. If you're eating with friends, make it a talking point if you like. Do a sensory deep-dive into your meal and use all your senses to experience the food and satisfy your body and mind.
6. Take small bites and put down the utensils when you are mindfully chewing your food. Give your body time to do its job.
7. Take the whole process slow. If you are generally busy, try to make time for at least one mindful eating session a day. It's like meditating, except you are nourishing your body and your mind.

You've probably noticed that many of the mindful eating principles are the same as intuitive eating principles. This is why the mindful eating approach is so helpful to create that peaceful and open mindset where you discover that food is your ally and not your enemy, and that you are not restricted as long as you listen to your body (Harvard Health Publishing, 2016).

Principle 8: Make Peace With Food

Making peace with food means giving yourself unconditional permission to eat what you want when your body needs it. This doesn't mean that you can't eat things that you usually enjoy like chocolate chip cookies or your favorite ice cream; intuitive eating just teaches you that you don't have to binge or overeat because when you are in that state of wellbeing, it won't make your body feel good, and you won't feel the need to. Food is not your enemy, and you don't have to cut any foods out of your life to be healthy and happy. Deprivation is the source of all evils when it comes to disordered eating patterns and overeating. On the other hand, making peace with food doesn't necessarily justify hedonistic hunger either—it's about finding your balance, being healthy, and feeling comfortable in your own body. Avoid the deprivation-binge pendulum which swings between two extremes: starving and depriving yourself or bingeing and overeating. If you let this pendulum gain momentum, it will not be able to stop in the middle, which is listening and acting on your body's natural cues (Rumsey, 2019).

Chapter 9: Understand the Eating 'Personalities' to Become an Intuitive Eater

Is everyone naturally an intuitive eater, or does everyone have the natural potential to become an intuitive eater? Well, we were all born intuitive eaters, but as we made our way through life, some of us stayed that way and some of us changed. There are a plethora of reasons why you could've abandoned an intuitive way of eating, mostly due to external circumstances such as how you were brought up, your family's eating habits, your self-esteem, and even food preferences. Now, interestingly enough, as adults can be classified into four different categories of eating in terms of our behavior and approach, and only one of them is the intuitive eater. These four categories were born from dieticians Evelyn Tribole and Elise Resch's years of consulting with patients with the aim to help them develop an intuitive eating approach. The researchers realized that they had developed a different approach to food during their childhood through to their adolescence, and they are practicing that mindset as adults. The four categories of eaters these pioneering dieticians were able to identify in their scores of patients were the Professional Dieter, the Unconscious Eater, the Intuitive Eater, and the Careful Eater. Some of these profiles may sound very similar; for example, it sounds like the Careful Eater and Professional Dieter have a lot in common. They are, however, distinct in some very important ways. Let's look at the Intuitive Eater when being compared to the four other types identified by these dieticians.

The Professional Dieter

Do you subscribe to some of those YouTube channels where the content creator tries a new diet every week or month and does a 'reveal' video so you can see if the diet can work for you? Alternatively, you may be obsessed with pinning new diet ideas and tricks like drinking lemon-coconut-charcoal water to boards on your Pinterest account and watching "what I eat in a day" videos to get quick weight-loss tips. Whatever the case, if you are the professional dieter type, you are always on a diet or on a mission planning a new diet. Why, you might ask? Probably because the current miracle diet you are on or were on for two days did not work. The Professional Dieter is an expert in yo-yo dieting and is all too familiar with the "go on a diet, lose weight, put the weight back on, bingeing in between, and then going back to dieting out of desperation" cycle. There are some things all Professional Dieters know, and that is the basics or more advanced components of portion sizes, calorie counting, and maybe even a thing or two about macros. The professional dieter is on an eternal journey to lose weight by going on diets; however, the journey will remain eternal because the weight doesn't stay off.

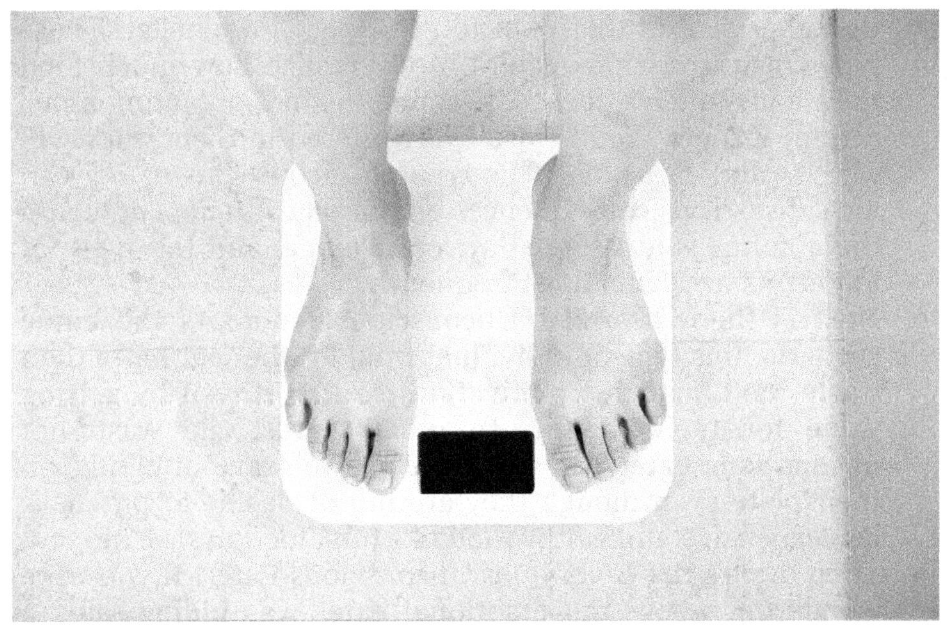

The Unconscious Eater

The Unconscious Eater is very much like the mindless eater, so in some sense, we've all been unconscious eaters. However, there are individuals who never pay any attention to what they are eating, and they are never fully conscious of the process while they're eating because they are always busy with something else. Even if it is just scrolling through social media on your phone while eating your lunch, this is a common example of unconscious eating; you really have no idea what's going into your mouth, what it tastes like exactly, how long you are taking to chew every bite, and sometimes even how much you've eaten. This eating personality is so prevalent that it's possible to distinguish between 4 different types of unconscious eaters.

- We'll begin by introducing our friend, the *Refuse-Not* Unconscious Eater. This type of unconscious eater will eat something because it is in their reach or even just in their presence. So they may be prepared to stand up and walk to the other side of the room to get a pig-in-a-blanket. These types of unconscious eaters rarely realize how much food they consume as it has become a kind of autonomous action; if there's food close by or offered to them, they will say yes and eat some. This type of unconscious eating can have disastrous consequences on one's health depending on the amount you eat per day, on average, and the types of foods that are eaten most frequently.

- Next is the *Waste-Not* Unconscious Eater. As the name suggests, this type of individual would rather eat more than waste food, and this motivation is often driven by getting value for their money. In other words, the waste-not unconscious eater can either refuse to leave anything on their plate even though they are full or decide to purchase less expensive, unhealthy food like junk food to save money.
- Then there's the *Emotional* Unconscious Eater. If you were wondering where the emotional eater was hiding, it is a subcategory of unconscious eating. Emotional Unconscious Eaters use eating to deal with issues that cause them emotional stress, to help them deal with loneliness, boredom, and anger. Emotional eaters learned somewhere in their life to find comfort in eating and to use it as a temporary solution for difficult emotional situations or feelings.
- The *Chaotic* Unconscious Eater is last on our list for no particular reason. This type of unconscious eater relates the most to the initial description—having the busiest day ever and eating whatever is the most convenient without putting too much thought into the nutritional side of things. This type of eater is so busy sometimes that they go for long stretches without eating and end up starved to the point of scarfing down three times as much as they would have normally.

These eaters are all victims of our information age and fast-paced lifestyles to some extent, and the one common factor that is absent in all of these situations is their full presence of mind while they are eating, like when you would be eating mindfully.

The Intuitive Eater

We are all well-versed in intuitive eating at this point, but let's go through the description and imprint it on our mind one more time—you know, deepen that neural pathway. If you are someone who relies on internal and physiological cues to base your food choices on and eat according to what and how much your body really needs, then you fit the profile of an Intuitive Eater. Intuitive Eaters won't force food down their throats if they don't like it, but they are aware of their bodies' nutritional requirements. They are unconditionally unapologetic about their food choices and eating habits because they put their bodies and minds first, and social norms and peer pressure second. Finally, an Intuitive Eater will completely reject any form of meal plan that puts them in a box, calorie counting that limits their food choices, as they see these as counterintuitive to what their body may need for nourishment.

The Careful Eater

Careful Eaters are not serial dieters, but they can be overly cautious about their food choices. They are well-educated when it comes to different food's sugar, fat, and sodium content, and they will first look at the nutritional contents of a product before buying it. A careful eater can also turn eating into an ethical or moral issue and decide to base their food choices on their ethical or moral beliefs. Eating unhealthy or not meeting general health standards can put a careful eater on a guilt-trip, and the first impression you would get from a careful eater is that they are concerned about healthy and organic eating. However, sometimes it's more about their bodies, body image and self-image, and the healthy eating approach can be a facade for weight-management (Habtemariam, 2019).

Creating Real Change

Being able to identify yourself among these different eating 'personalities' can have a profound and positive effect on your attempt to transition to intuitive eating because it provides insight into the components and eating habits you are currently struggling with the most. We are not always aware of subtle behaviors that can make a big difference in our overall approach to eating, and awareness and understanding help you to be more informed and prepared if you want to or need to make a mental and physical change. Some of us may also have realized that we can identify with more than one of these types and that some of us will have overlapping dominant characteristics. Knowing this is just as useful as identifying with only one type; if you know this information, you can use it to create change in your life. Let's look at the types again and see if there are some behaviors that can be changed for the better:

The Professional Dieter

If you've identified yourself as a Professional Dieter, you've probably noticed a few big differences between your habits and the habits of an Intuitive Eater, and even more so when it comes to the mindset. Your mindset is completely focused on food and eating even though you want that element in your life to have less influence—yet you've become kind of obsessed about everything related to food in a negative way because you've declared food to be your enemy. Where do we go from here? The best place to start is with your mindset. When you are confronted with food, try not to see it as bad or forbidden. Everything in moderation is acceptable. When you wake up in the morning, and your body is not hungry yet, don't eat the "boiled egg and cracker" from "Day 3" if you are not hungry yet. Give your body time. If you need to leave home, pack something or get something along the way when you start to feel hungry. Start listening to your body, and you will feel a weight coming off your shoulders. Remind yourself that you are not suddenly going to start eating everything you see, in contrast, you are only going to eat what your body needs.

The Careful Eater

If you are a Careful Eater, one of your positive traits is that you are deliberate about what you eat. However, you spend too much time thinking about it and deliberating nutritional choices where you could have let your body guide you. What your body needs is nutrition, so it will lead you towards eating foods that contain the nutritional components it requires. Try to do less label reading. If organic is important, make sure you do your shopping at a store that sells organic produce. However, don't deny your body anything because if you do, it's just another form of restrictive eating or dieting. Allow yourself to be free and to enjoy everything in life. Have you been truly enjoying yourself lately? Health is not only physical but also a mental component in your life, and if your body is MSG-free but you're still not feeling fulfilled, there might be a puzzle piece missing, and its name is probably fun! Try something new and take your tastebuds on an adventure. Spend time with friends and relax about what you are eating and drinking—your body will tell you when you've had enough.

Gather Round All Unconscious Eaters

All unconscious eaters have one major thing in common, and this is that they do not pay attention when they eat or to what they are eating. In some cases, they are also not very mindful of why they are eating, and they don't rely on their bodies to help them regulate their need for nourishment. For unconscious eaters, the starting point is paying attention, being present every time they eat, and learning to tune with their bodies. For example, when you are stressed because you have an important meeting in an hour and you feel like having a muffin from the cafeteria, does your body want that muffin if you just had breakfast two hours ago? Your tummy may fool you by grumbling. However, if you know that the primary reason you want that muffin is that you want to self-medicate to ease your soaring stress levels, then it's time to reassess the situation and try another way to safely and effectively deal with stress and anxiety. A productive approach is to prepare yourself for the workday before you actually go to work by meditating, reading, or stretching your body to get out unnecessary tension. You can also reflect on your day and keep a diary. Try a variety of things, and when you have that urge to eat for any other reason except for hunger, stop yourself, remove yourself from the situation, and have a discussion.

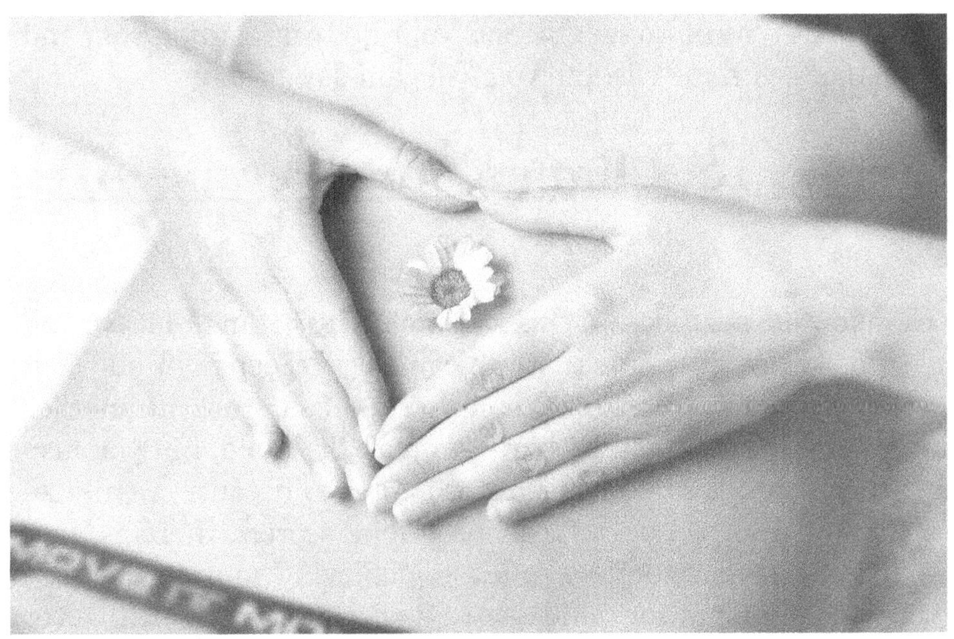

Principle 9: Honor Your Hunger

Hunger is one of your body's ways of telling you that it needs nourishment. If you are in touch with your body, you will know when it is really hungry and when it is just craving something. We now know that hunger isn't always hunger and that even though you have unconditional freedom as an intuitive eater, you can benefit from managing hunger if you know that you're going to be attending social events or other gatherings that are based on eating. It's never a good idea to starve yourself. If you are going to try and ignore sensations of true hunger, your body is going to react by making you completely ravenous. Many intuitive eaters are people who like to take one or two bites from something or order a really small portion because that's all their body needs at that moment to satisfy their hunger. No one is the same physiologically, but a "starting from small" approach is a great way to honor your hunger and make sure you don't overeat and fall back into the dieting cycle again. Pay attention to when you are hungry, what type of hunger signals your body is sending you, and analyze them with the wisdom you will gain day-to-day.

Chapter 10: Change Your Perspective

To change your perspective, this final chapter is going to leave you with some key components that you can always keep in mind when it comes to intuitive eating. When you've been stuck in another routine for so long, it can be hard to break the mold, but you also may experience times where you don't want to because we all like our comfort zones. One of the best-kept secrets there is that breaking out of your comfort zone and achieving your goals is one of the most liberating and satisfying things you will ever experience in your life, and it will make you a stronger, more resilient individual. Here are your practical takeaways for a great start to your best health and your best year yet!

Reject the Diet Mentality

Diet culture is all of those restrictive external focuses that keeps you trapped in a cycle of chaos and a forced sense of control. A healing diet mentality, like intuitive eating, requires you to return your sense of control to an internal place, and this starts with learning to practice self-awareness and unconditional non-judgment. It is easy to write down, but if your brain has been wired a certain way for years, it can be hard to change. It's important to be patient and kind to yourself when you encounter obstacles in your self-awareness journey as this journey of getting to know yourself again will be part of your intuitive eating journey all the way.

Helpful Activities

Here are some questions you can ask yourself, and answer truthfully when diet culture gets the most of you:

- Has dieting or following diet culture ever helped me to reach my long-term goals or help me to trust myself around food?
- Why is diet culture suddenly getting the most of me? Can I identify the trigger?
- If you can't find the answer immediately, let the thought linger at the back of your mind. It'll come to you.

Make Peace With Food

Being in a love-hate relationship with a substance that is primarily supposed to keep you alive and healthy can be exhausting and extremely frustrating. If you've been restricting yourself or relying on any other external food rules, food is more likely your enemy than your friend, which means that there is no freedom or unconditional acceptance in this relationship. Making peace with food is a crucial component of reconnecting with your inner intuitive eating self and rekindling your relationship with your body and that which gives you sustenance.

Helpful Activity

- Write down all the foods that you think are forbidden or just generally a "no-no."
- Choose one item from your list.

- Go to the grocery store and buy the forbidden item. Take note of how you feel when the shop assistant swipes it past the sensor and it goes "ping!"
- Keep it in your fridge until a time where you are alone, mildly hungry, and dish some up for yourself.
- Eat your forbidden food mindfully and focus all your sense on the food. Also, focus on the emotional experience you connect to eating this food and whether you have any sense of enjoyment.
- Put your findings in writing and reflect on your experience.

Honor Your Hunger

Hunger is supposed to be a biologically driven instinct, so it's fascinating to think that we've succeeded in completely bypassing its primary function, which is to keep us healthy and find other, unhealthy ways in the quest to find the ultimate level of health. How ironic. Ignoring or manipulating your own hunger does not set you up to look after one of your most fundamental needs and sends a message to yourself that self-care is not important. Real hunger also comes from internal signals and not external or societal signals like "one o'clock means it's lunchtime." Because of the way society is structured, we are prone to rely on external structures, which can cause us to eat when our bodies do not need food.

Helpful Activities

- Take a day and focus on what drives your hunger. Is it:
    1. Emotions or boredom?
    2. A specific time?
    3. A habitual food date with a friend?

4. When food is nearby?
5. Or, when your energy levels, stomach, and ability to focus are starting to falter?

Which one is the best way to honor your hunger?

Discover the Satisfaction Factor

Do all your eating experiences satisfy you, or only some? If you've been following a diet, restricting your food or calorie intake in other ways, or adhering to the requests of the food pushers or guilt trips of the food police, then you likely have a low satisfaction level because your eating choices have not been coming from inside yourself. You have the unconditional freedom to savor all of your eating experiences of which you make the choices. Your level of enjoyment is likely connected on a deeper level to how focused you are on the eating process, and this process can start as early as when you think about what you want to make for dinner tonight. If you are satisfied with food on an internal level, you are less likely to follow external and restrictive guidelines that are not beneficial for your health or happiness.

Helpful Activities

- Ditch the diet and plan your own menu based on foods you enjoy.
- If some of the foods are usually forbidden, try to incorporate them one at a time into your new menu.
- Go shopping for your ingredients and remember to include your forbidden food.

- Throw yourself into the whole process, from cooking to eating, enjoy and savor your food, stop when you are full, and reflect on the difference between this experience and eating when you are on a diet.

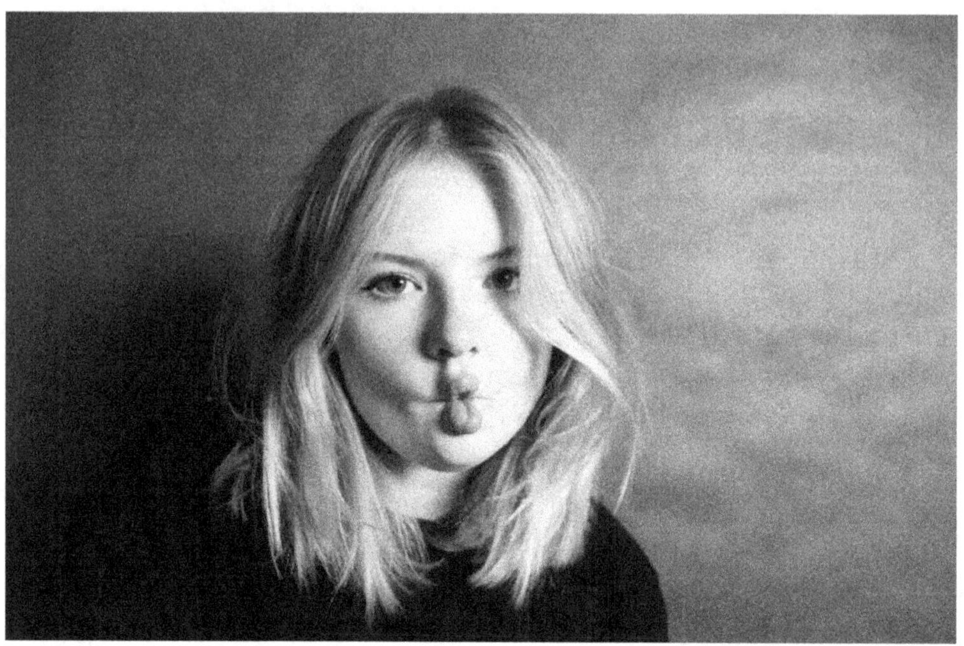

Feel Your Fullness

At the very center of the feeling your fullness principle is having respect for your body's limits. This respect is deeply rooted in knowing that it's okay for you to stop when you do because you know you have unconditional permission to eat again when you feel hungry, whether it's in five minutes or five hours, and also because you know your body has limits when it comes to how much food it actually needs. Eating, then, also requires that full-body presence or mindfulness so you have a deep sense of awareness of when your body becomes full. Otherwise, you won't be able to recognize when it's time to stop eating if you are either distracted or unconsciously eating. So, what can you do?

Helpful Activities

- When you start eating mindfully, it's easier to become aware of that sense of fullness. However, that doesn't always mean you always stop when you need to. So, the next time you realize that you've consumed more than your body needs, ask yourself some questions to clarify the situation:
    1. Did you overeat because you weren't fully present while you were eating?
    2. Did you feel anxious because you didn't know when your next meal will be?
    3. Did you enjoy the food so much that you struggled to stop eating?
- If you answered yes to any of these questions, it can be a learning experience for you to focus on your body the next time you eat something. Just remember to be kind to yourself and not be harsh because you "did something wrong" or "made a mistake." Kindness is part of intuitive eating.
- Pro tip: When you feel that first sensation of fullness, put down your utensils and give yourself about a minute to let the food settle. Then, based on how your body feels, you can decide whether you've had enough based on the cues your body gives you.

Challenge the Food Police

The food police are all the voices in your head and around you that are feeding you toxic information about eating, food types, and body image. The food police can be anyone, including yourself, and toxic information includes anything that doesn't appreciate your unconditional freedom to choose what you want to eat, when you want to eat, and respecting your body's needs. The informative food police will give you or base their opinions on will always be derived from sources that are externally controlled like diet culture and an outlook that does not support individuality. These messages spread negativity, and if you have your own personal food police in your head, it's time to get rid of that little but loud voice.

Helpful Activities

- Keeping tabs of how many food police run-ins you experience in a day can provide you with a clearer picture of what you are up against. These experiences include your own inner food police and external experiences.
- If you know that you have your own squad policing your thoughts, assess their influence. Do they have power over your choices or are you pushing them to the background?
- Practice standing up for yourself and talking back to that voice. It's about time it receives a talking-to.
- Give yourself a vocabulary assessment by focusing on how many times you use the word "should" when you talk about food. This suggests that you have a restrictive mentality and think that some foods are allowed but some are not.

Emotions Do Not Equal Eating

For many of us, food is one of the few sources of comfort when we go through a painful or stressful period in our lives. Comfort eating, in principle, isn't unethical or wrong. The problem comes in when you experience the after-effects of shame and guilt following a food coma, which is unhealthy for your mind, and the fact that emotional eating is unhealthy for your body. Food has different connections for everybody; for example, for most of us, food is a way to come together in a social way. If we can focus on and respect the positive aspects of emotional eating, which would be celebrating, honoring a memory, or coming together as a family or a group of friends, then it is possible to celebrate with food in a healthy way instead of using it to try and numb overwhelming feelings.

Helpful Activity

- Think of an emotional eating experience—a time when you ate purely for the pleasure of the food or because you felt a positive emotional connection.
- Now, think of a time when you also ate because of emotions, but because they were painful and you were trying to numb the pain.
- Think about eating to cope with emotions as only one choice you have within a sea of other, more productive choices you can make to deal productively with your pain. Can you identify a few?
- Which choices would you want to make instead of eating next time you experience hardship in your life?

Honor Your Health With Gentle Nutrition

Intuitive eating is one of the most beautiful ways to honor your health, even though diet culture may disagree with you. The idea of

Intuitive eating is solidly based on practicing self-acceptance and self-care. This is the type of self-care that finds its roots in the ability to nurture and identify your physical and mental needs on a constant basis. Being able to do this effectively does require being flexible and, as we've seen throughout the book, being able to adapt to different, non-intuitive eating-friendly environments. By gently focusing on providing your body the nutrition it needs while satisfying yourself as a whole being will keep you at an optimal level of physical and mental health. As you enjoy eating, focus on adding nutrition in a way you like. If you are focused on being fulfilled, healthy additions will come naturally. If you need to ease into it, take it day by day.

Helpful Advice

- Write down your favorite healthy foods like fruits, vegetables, and unprocessed carbs.
- Now, write down your favorite foods you primarily like because they are tasty, nice to cook with, and fun or nice to eat.
- After writing down your two lists, combine them and create one list, focusing on how you can use some of these items together to create tasty meals.
- Try out and experiment using some healthy ingredients with some of your favorite ones in meals and cook them the way you like them.
- Enjoy!

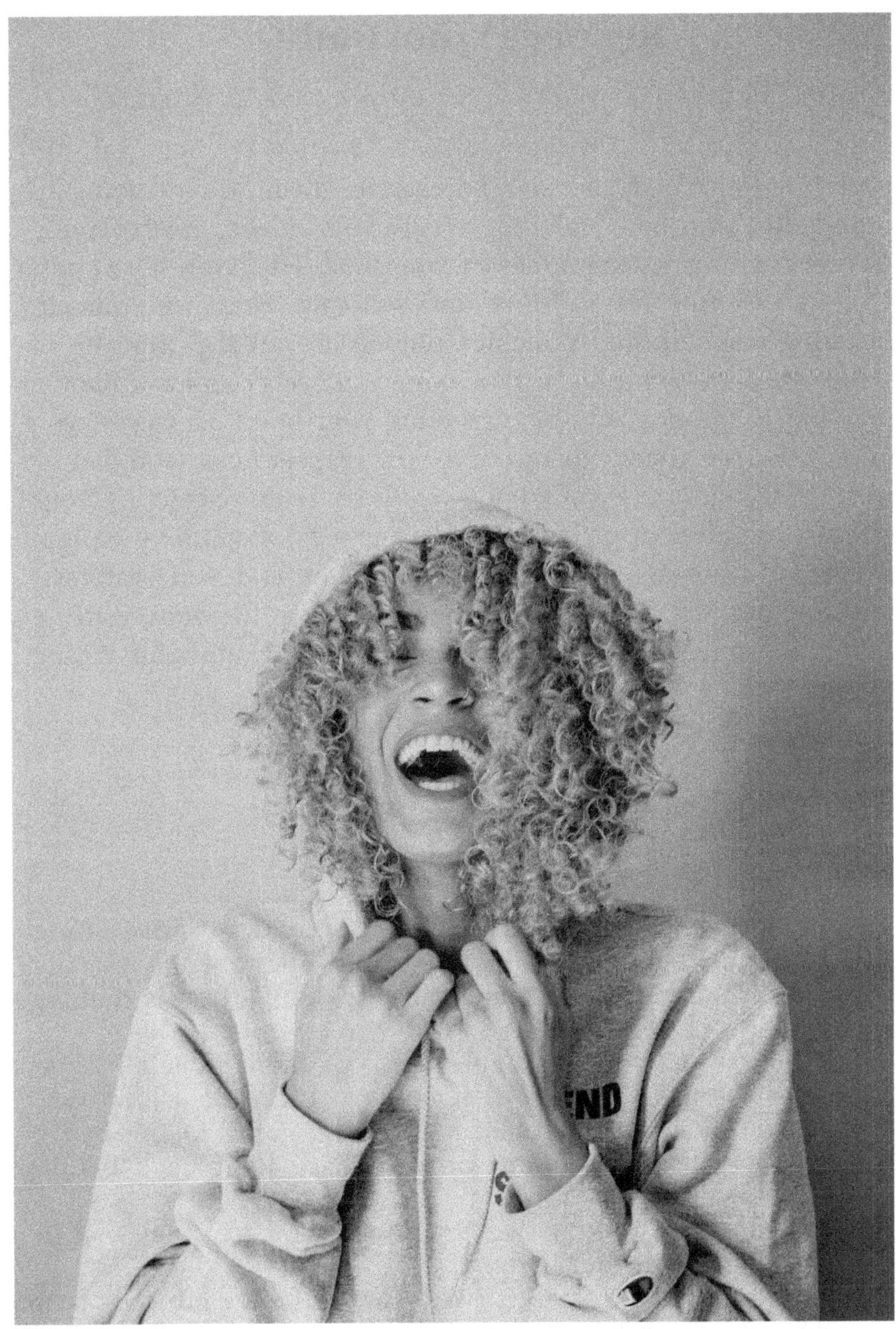

Respect Your Body

Respecting your body doesn't necessarily mean you're going to instantly like your body, fall in love with your thighs, or stop trying different contouring techniques on your nose. However, it's a start, and it is essential for self-love and self-care. Starving yourself, restricting yourself, and policing yourself are all the opposite of having respect for your body. Punishing yourself because you had a candy bar is the opposite of respecting your body. However, you can grow to love your body out of having respect for it, and just by realizing how amazing your body really is. Truly respecting your body also requires applying all the principles of intuitive eating: savoring your meals, honoring your hunger and your fullness, drowning out the food police, enjoying your freedom, getting quality movement, and having healthy and meaningful eating experiences.

Helpful Advice

- Okay, let's focus on our bodies for a second. Intuitive eating is all about the inside, but we do have an outside and the reason many of us get caught in the dieting trap is that we want to change the way we look.
- The first and very valid question is: is there an activity you are no longer interested in doing because of a low body image? For many people, it could be going to the beach because they don't want others to see them in a bikini. What's yours?
- Do you want to stay like this, or do you feel the need to reconnect with your body?
- Is there an outfit you can wear that flatters your body that you can wear to this event and that you will feel more confident in?

- Finally, if you don't want to go all the way, can the activity be modified so you can still enjoy it but without feeling exposed?

Feel the Difference With Movement

This is the final principle in the book, as well as the final one in this chapter. Exercise is healthy, but some have a misperception of how much exercise they need and what the definition of exercise is, so they stay away from it. Movement can be a better term than exercise because exercise is not necessarily what keeps your body healthy, it can be what keeps it moving. Movement means keeping your body busy, but not necessarily doing a full weights training session at the gym. Some people prefer working out and exercising, as it has many benefits and gives you a mental kick, but movement can be just as beneficial. When it comes to the principles of intuitive eating, you should be free to do what you enjoy, as long as you recognize the benefits of movement. Exercising sessions like aerobics or dance classes or even HIIT are associated with diet culture, but this is one component that is beneficial for your body and that can help to keep your heart healthy and keep that sense of longevity.

Helpful Tips:

- What is the first thought that pops into your head when you think about the words 'movement' or 'exercise?'
- Is movement something that you see as restrictive or the kind of activity that can clear your mind and keep you fit and healthy?

- Make a list of all the types of movements and exercises you can think of. Which ones look most appealing?
- Try out the one that looks most enjoyable, and focus on enjoying the experience. Feel what is happening in your body, and make a note of how you feel after you completed the movement (Yeiter, 2017).

This is your intuitive eating workbook. Take it, enjoy it, and learn to be unconditionally free, healthy from the inside out, and the happiest you have ever been. Use the exercises to make yourself wiser, and never judge yourself for past behaviors, reactions, or what you may see as 'mistakes.'

Conclusion

This is intuitive eating. It is not a monolithic idea, but a multifaceted one filled with possibilities, creativity, individuality, positivity, and love. Self-love. Caring about yourself and your body is what's most important. However, for those of us who have been creating those neural pathways that promote restrictive eating habits and calorie-counting, this may be a challenging process. The first step is to recognize the benefits of intuitive eating. The world still needs to wake up to this type of freedom, and because the idea of freedom has been turned completely upside down by diet culture, this may take a while. However, a few pioneers in the quest for self-acceptance, self-care, and unconditional happiness and freedom can make a difference for those around them that struggle with crippling self-doubt, food-related guilt, and unnecessary self-criticism.

A key starting point is to identify when in your life you stopped being an intuitive eater. Because intuitive eating focuses on mental and physical health, understanding yourself and where your triggers come from is essential for freeing yourself from them and accepting food instead of hating it.

This is my challenge to you. I challenge you to create your own happiness, because I wish you happiness. To reach fulfillment, self-acceptance, and freedom in life can be a journey riddled with obstacles. If you see each obstacle as an opportunity to learn and embrace it with open arms, you will reach your highest level of freedom, wisdom, and experience in life. In our lifetime, dealing with food and food issues are in many cases some of our biggest struggles in life, and they shouldn't be. It should be easy to eat, and it should be enjoyable. It should be part of your self-care routine. Embrace yourself, learn from your previous restrictive thought patterns, move with joy, and spread the love so others can see how living with an unconditional relationship towards food and eating can bring out the best in you and those around you.

If you need to start at the beginning, do so with confidence. This is your guide, your knowledge, and you can use it to gain your own wisdom. As long as you appreciate life, appreciate food, and appreciate who you are, unconditionally, and be kind to yourself and others, always. That is intuitive eating.

References

Altindas, D. (2021). *Photo by Deniz Altindas on Unsplash.*
Unsplash.com.

https://unsplash.com/photos/t1XLQvDqt_4

Andrea Hardy. (2019, November 4). *The psychological
consequences of diets.* Ignite Nutrition.
https://ignitenutrition.ca/blog/why-diets-dont-work-the-
psychological-impacts-of-dieting/

Ascenzo, M. (2021). *Photo by Mattia Ascenzo on Unsplash.*
Unsplash.com. https://unsplash.com/photos/thW2sk-646E

Billie. (2021). Body image. In *Unsplash.*
https://unsplash.com/photos/k2vn6he4lDQ

Bjarnadottir, A. (2019, June 19). *Mindful eating 101 — A
beginner's guide.* Healthline.
https://www.healthline.com/nutrition/mindful-eating-
guide#intro

Brocchi, L. (2021). Imperfect. In *Unsplash.*
https://unsplash.com/photos/5SxSmTfJYc4

Cajina, I. (2021). *Photo by Ivana Cajina on Unsplash.*
Unsplash.com. https://unsplash.com/photos/dnL6ZIpht2s

Comas, J. (2015, July 8). *Grace under (food) pressure: 5 effective strategies for handling food pushers*. Girls Gone Strong. https://www.girlsgonestrong.com/blog/articles/food-pushers/

Compton, C. (2020, June 9). *Breaking up with diet culture.* The Alliance for Eating Disorders Awareness. https://www.allianceforeatingdisorders.com/breaking-up-with-diet-culture/

Dooley, I. (2021). Ice cream. In *Unsplash.* https://unsplash.com/photos/TLD6iCOlyb0

Dutta, S. S. (2019, September 22). *What is intuitive eating and is it healthy?* News-Medical.net. https://www.news-medical.net/health/What-is-Intuitive-Eating-and-Is-It-Healthy.aspx#:~:text=Studies%20have%20found%20that%20intuitive

Habtemariam, A. (2019, July 15). *The four eating personalities.* Truly Real Nutrition. https://www.trulyrealnutrition.com/blog/2019/7/15/the-four-eating-personalities#:~:text=Intuitive%20eaters%20make%20foo d%20choices

Harvard Health Publishing. (2016, January 16). *8 steps to mindful eating - Harvard Health*. Harvard Health; Harvard Health. https://www.health.harvard.edu/staying-healthy/8-steps-to-mindful-eating

Holbrook, S. (2020, December 30). *Intuitive eating is a happier and healthier way to eat—here's how to begin*. Real Simple. https://www.realsimple.com/health/nutrition-diet/healthy-eating/intuitive-eating

Iven, W. (2021). *Photo by William Iven on Unsplash*. Unsplash.com. https://unsplash.com/photos/SpVHcbuKi6E

Jennings, K.-A. (2019, June 25). *A quick guide to intuitive eating*. Healthline; Healthline Media. https://www.healthline.com/nutrition/quick-guide-intuitive-eating

Korodetz, N. (2017, March 24). *Diet culture and our relationship with food*. Nicole Korodetz.

https://nicolekorodetzrd.com/diet-culture-relationship-food/

Kraft, K. (2021). *Photo by Kenzie Kraft on Unsplash.* Unsplash.com.

https://unsplash.com/photos/Oh81uk8CoEA

Lark, B. (2021). *Photo by Brooke Lark on Unsplash.* Unsplash.com.

https://unsplash.com/photos/AgD6OBNXF0Q

Lysenko, M. (2021). *Photo by Maria Lysenko on Unsplash.* Unsplash.com.

https://unsplash.com/photos/mjaMxrxNMHY

Mayer, M. (2021). Girl Eating. In *Unsplash.* https://unsplash.com/photos/VxdzpgSrqmg

Mayo Clinic Staff. (2021). *Can mindfulness exercises help me?* Mayo Clinic. https://www.mayoclinic.org/healthy-lifestyle/consumer-health/in-depth/mindfulness-exercises/art-20046356#:~:text=Mindfulness%20is%20a%20type%20of

McGinley, K. (2017, June 22). *5 ways to embrace imperfection.* Chopra. https://chopra.com/articles/5-ways-to-embrace-imperfection

Miller, S. G. (2016, April). *The science of hunger: How to control it and fight cravings*. Livescience.com; Live Science. https://www.livescience.com/54248-controlling-your-hunger.html

Norwood Themes. (2021). *Photo by NordWood Themes on Unsplash*. Unsplash.com. https://unsplash.com/photos/vx7JmlGDSX4

Owens, J. (2021). *Photo by Jakob Owens on Unsplash*. Unsplash.com. https://unsplash.com/photos/SaO8RBYCobs

Petre, A. (2020, April 2). *What to know about orthorexia*. Healthline. https://www.healthline.com/nutrition/orthorexia-nervosa-101#what-is-orthorexia

Rumsey, A. (2019, June 14). *What is intuitive eating and how is it different from mindful eating?* Alissa Rumsey Nutrition | New York Registered Dietitian Nutritionist | Virtual Intuitive Eating Coaching. https://alissarumsey.com/intuitive-eating/what-is-intuitive-eating/

Siora Photography. (2021). Measuring tape. In *Unsplash*. https://unsplash.com/photos/cixohzDpNIo

The Original Intuitive Eating Pros. (2021). *Studies*. Intuitive Eating. https://www.intuitiveeating.org/resources/studies/#:~:text=Women%20with%20high%20Intuitive%20Eating

Xen and the Art of Mindful Eating. (2016, December 6). *7 easy tips to deal with "friendly" food pushers*. Xen and the Art of Mindful Eating. https://www.theartofmindfuleating.com/7-easy-tips-to-deal-with-friendly-food-pushers/

Yeiter, J. (2017, November 24). *Intuitive eating principles: With activities*. Healwithjill. https://www.healwithjill.com/post/2017/11/24/intuitive-eating-principles-with-activities